Understanding
Depression

Nigel Lester, M.D.

Kwame McKenzie, M.D.

Family Doctor Books

IMPORTANT
This book is intended not as a substitute for personal medical advice but as a supplement to that advice for the patient who wishes to understand more about his or her condition.

Before taking any form of treatment
YOU SHOULD ALWAYS CONSULT YOUR MEDICAL PRACTITIONER.

In particular (without limit) you should note that advances in medical science occur rapidly and some information about drugs and treatment contained in this booklet may very soon be out of date.

ISBN 10: 1-4285-0004-9
ISBN 13: 978-1-4285-0004-4

Contents

About the authors

Dr. Nigel Lester
Dr. Lester has worked as a Psychiatrist in both the United States and Great Britain. He is a former Director of the Mental Health Program for the department of HIV Medicine at St Vincent's Hospital in New York City and Attending Psychiatrist at Northern Westchester Hospital in Mount Kisco, New York. He has a special interest in promoting better understanding of mental health issues amongst the public and other medical professionals.

Dr. Kwame McKenzie
Dr. McKenzie is a Senior Lecturer and Consultant Psychiatrist at the Royal Free Hospital and University College Medical School, London, England. He is committed to improving the understanding of mental illness and has written over 200 articles, hosted a TV series, and conducted numerous radio interviews on the subject.

Introduction

What is depression?

We all have low moods from time to time. For instance, if a relationship breaks up we may feel shocked, we may cry, not feel like eating, get mad and irritable, sleep poorly, and become tetchy and anxious. Usually, the mood passes after a few days and we get back to our normal way of living. We may say that we have been "depressed," sad, or have "had the blues."

But low moods like this are not what doctors call depression. Instead, they use the term to describe a more severe illness that a person has had for at least a few weeks, affecting the body as well as the mind. Depression can begin for no reason at all and may sometimes be life-threatening. No one symptom indicates whether you have just a low mood or what some people call "clinical depression." Many of the symptoms are similar; however, when you are depressed, they are usually more intense and continue for longer.

A simple rule of thumb is that, if your low mood affects all parts of your life, lasts for two weeks or more, or brings you to the point of thinking about suicide, you should seek help. Try to remember that depression is an illness that can be treated and you will feel better in time.

Many people with depression are worried about talking to their primary care physician because they believe he or she will think it a sign of weakness. But family doctors have years of experience in dealing with depression. They will listen to you sympathetically and can refer you to a psychiatrist if necessary. Psychiatrists are specialists who have specific experience in the diagnosis and treatment of depression. They may prescribe medication, but will probably also tell you about self-help organizations, counseling, and psychotherapy or relaxation techniques. You may get advice on ways of decreasing your stress or coming to terms with bereavement or other loss. Your family doctor and psychiatrist will be a mine of information.

But if you do not feel that you can talk to your doctor at first, talk with a friend. You will be surprised how many people have experience of depression either first hand or because they know someone who has been depressed. They may be able to give you support and advice but, even if they just listen, talking to someone usually helps.

How common is depression?

Many famous people have suffered from depression, including Abraham Lincoln, Queen Victoria, and Winston Churchill, who called depression his "black dog."

Many writers and actors have suffered from depression and the author William Styron wrote a book about his depressive illness, entitled *Darkness Visible*.

Facts about depression

- At least one in five adults will suffer from depression in their lifetime.
- In any given one-year period, nearly 1 in 10 of the population, or about 18.8 million American adults, suffer from a depressive illness.
- Depression affects all age groups.
- Women are diagnosed as suffering from it twice as often as men.
- Depression is very treatable.

The rates of depression have increased over the last 40 years, which may be the result of the way we live our lives now. For many people, the world is becoming increasingly stressful and stress can lead to depression. Stress factors include increases in divorce rates and crime rates, longer working hours for some and unemployment for others are just some of the factors that make life a strain for those affected.

Where we live may be important for our risk of depression too. One study suggested that people who live in an inner-city area are twice as likely to be depressed as those who live in rural locations. Although it has proved difficult to find an exact reason for this, it is clear that the environment is important to the risk of depression.

The good news is that no matter what the cause of depression, it can be treated and treated effectively. Most people who are depressed and get treatment get better.

KEY POINTS

■ Low moods are thought of as depression if they persist and affect all parts of your life

■ Depression is common

■ Depression can be treated effectively

What is depression?

An illness of mind and body

Depression is an illness of mind and body. Most people have both physical and psychological symptoms, but their exact nature will vary from one person to another. Different symptoms will be more or less prominent in each person's illness. Some people report no symptoms at all but begin behaving in an unusual way—for example, one previously law-abiding woman who came to my clinic had started shop-lifting when she became depressed.

Psychological symptoms
Low mood

Despite the use of the label "depression," not everyone with this illness feels low. Some are anxious, some say they are emotionally numb, and some have no mood changes but come to their doctor with unexplained physical symptoms or with a change in behavior.

Low mood in depression is much more intense than the way you feel when you are disappointed or just

Symptoms of depression

Depression has a wide range of possible psychological and physical symptoms. What one person experiences as symptoms of depression may well be very different from what another person experiences.

Psychological

- Low mood
- Loss of interest in things you used to enjoy
- Anxiety
- Emotional numbness
- Depressive thinking
- Concentration and memory problems
- Delusions
- Hallucinations
- Suicidal impulse

Physical

- Sleep problems—difficulty getting to sleep, waking up early, or sleeping too much
- Mental and physical slowing down
- Increase or decrease in appetite
- Increase or decrease in weight
- Loss of interest in sex
- Tiredness
- Constipation
- Menstrual period irregularities

upset. It is a persistent feeling of sadness, emptiness, loss, and dread. Some say it is like living with a cloud over you and it takes over every part of your life.

Diurnal variations
In moderate or severe depression, low mood is often worse in the morning and improves slightly during the day—though it never goes away. This is called diurnal variation.

Anhedonia
Low mood makes it impossible to enjoy anything and you may even lose interest in your hobbies. Nothing brings you pleasure. Doctors call this symptom anhedonia.

In some milder depressions, low mood may be worse in the evenings than in the mornings and there may be the odd good day. However, the bad ones outnumber the good. If depression is mild you may be able to enjoy other people's company—though without stimulation you will soon become disenchanted again.

With the low mood comes a tendency to weep more often at the slightest upset or even with no upset at all.

Anxiety
When we feel threatened, a hormone called adrenaline is released and blood is directed to our muscles and brain so that we can think quickly and flee if we need to. We feel on edge, jumpy, and tense but, if nothing happens, the feeling passes in a few minutes. In someone who is depressed, these anxious feelings can last for months.

Some people wake in the morning in a state of high anxiety because they dread the day ahead. Anxiety can outweigh low mood and be the most prominent symptom in depression. If you are in a state of anxiety you may find that you get irritable and snap a lot which is obviously difficult for other people to live with as well as for you.

Emotional numbness
Some people who are severely depressed say that they feel like they have completely lost their emotions and this is one of the most distressing symptoms of depression. You feel numb. You can't cry and you feel like there are no tears left. You may not feel that you are part of the world because you do not think that you have feelings. You may feel distant and unfeeling about even people very close to you such as your partner, family. or children.

Depressive thinking

Your thinking changes when you are suffering from depression. You see the world differently and everything appears in a negative light. This distorted view simply reinforces the depression.

You may blame yourself for unfortunate events more than you should while not allowing yourself to take credit for things that you have done well. The good things that you have done throughout your life are forgotten and the bad are vividly remembered and blown up out of all proportion.

You may find yourself concentrating on the negative detail and ignoring the bigger picture. To take an extreme example, someone who had passed an exam

Depressive thinking

Depressive thinking makes a person see the world in a negative light. There are three elements to depressive thinking:

1. Negative thoughts, for example, "I am a failure at work"

2. High, unreasonable expectations, for example, "I cannot be happy unless everyone likes me and thinks I am good at my job"

3. Mistakes in thinking, for example:
   (a) jumping to negative conclusions
   (b) focusing on negative details of a situation and ignoring the good parts
   (c) coming to a general conclusion on the basis of a single incident
   (d) coming to the conclusion that things that are nothing to do with you are your fault

with 99 percent might ignore the good result and concentrate on the one percent that they had gotten wrong.

You may also start jumping to negative conclusions and jumping to general conclusions from single events.

For instance, a fashion model I once treated thought that she was ugly and everyone hated her because a man who passed her in the street gave her a weird look.

These sorts of negative thinking patterns undermine you. They lead to worry, a lack of confidence, and feelings of worthlessness, and your world becomes full of gloomy thoughts, self-doubt, and anxieties. As a result, you feel more depressed or anxious and so a vicious circle is set up.

Case history: Carrie

Carrie is a secretary; her boss is late catching the train and on his way out, he says, "Could you type this report up for me, I have made a few corrections." Carrie is depressed, and because of this she thinks she is a failure. She believes that she has to correct the report because she is bad at her job. She becomes more depressed because she has the unreasonable expectation that she must be perfect in her job if she is to enjoy her life.

In reality, she is good at her job but she doesn't think so. She concentrates on little things that go wrong rather than the big things that go right. She forgets the fact that she was given a pay raise because her company values her so much. She also ignores the fact that her boss is known to be indecisive and always changes reports that he has written. She concentrates on the negative details and jumps to a general conclusion based on a single incident—this makes her depressed.

While she is typing the report another thought comes to her: "Could the boss be late because he had to correct my sloppy work? If the deal falls through it will be all my fault!" She blames herself for things that are not her fault, and this fuels her depression.

Concentration and memory problems

If you are consumed by worries and depressive thoughts, it can be difficult to think about anything else. You may find it hard to concentrate and this leads to problems. You have to concentrate on something to remember it, so it is not surprising that poor concentration and memory problems go together. Problems with concentration also lead to indecision and inattention; you may feel muddled and confused. These feelings can be so severe as to be mistaken for dementia.

Delusions and hallucinations
Delusions

If you should become severely depressed, your thinking can become so distorted that you lose touch with reality. Your mind can start playing tricks on you and you may even fear that you are going insane. You are not; you are severely depressed and will get better with treatment. Delusions can occur in severe depression; thankfully, they are rare (because they are so distressing).

A delusion is a false belief that is held unshakably by the person who has it. In depression, delusions reflect and reinforce the depressed mood. This happened with James whom I treated some time ago. He believed that he should give himself up to the police because by mistake, he had left a store without paying for an apple five years previously. He thought that the police were looking for him and that there was no way out. He believed that he had brought shame on his family and was worthless. It was impossible to make him believe that he was not public enemy number one, that anyone can make a mistake and that no one would be bothered about it.

Others believe that they are the wickedest person in the world or that people want to get rid of them because they are so bad. Some people believe that they have no money at all, others that they are decaying or even that they are dead. There are as many different types of delusion as there are ideas in the human mind but all of them reflect the depressed mood and depressive thinking.

Hallucinations
Whereas delusions are false thoughts, hallucinations involve perceiving things that are not real—usually sounds. For example, some severely depressed people hear voices when there is no one there. The voices sound like people in the room talking to them and are frighteningly real. The voices may criticize them or tell them that they are wicked. The voices reinforce the depression. Some people see or smell things that are not there but this is rarer.

Suicidal impulses
When you are in the depths of depression the past looks bad and full of mistakes, the present is awful, and you dread the future. Some come to the conclusion that life is not worth living, that everyone

would be better off without them and that they should take their own life.

Many depressed people think about suicide—even if it is just a passing thought. Many do not actually contemplate committing suicide but go to bed at night hoping that they will not wake up, and so get away from the terrible torture of living.

Most people decide that they can't do it, perhaps because it would be too drastic, or the effect it would have on their family, or because of religious beliefs. Some people come to the conclusion that they have not done it because they are cowards and this makes them feel even more ashamed and depressed.

If you think about suicide you are at risk of committing it. Get help urgently: see your doctor, go to the emergency room, or call a hotline. Depression can be treated.

Physical symptoms

Depression can cause a number of physical symptoms. Those people affected often come to the conclusion that they have a physical illness because they feel so tired and off-color or are in pain.

Sleep problems

Sleep problems are common in depression and are sometimes partially to blame for the tiredness that may be experienced. If you are suffering from a moderate or severe depression you may wake up in the morning hours earlier than usual and then find it impossible to get back to sleep. All depressed people can find it difficult to get to sleep because they worry and may suffer from broken nights—waking up a number of times before the morning.

Mental and physical slowing

If you are depressed, you may feel like a machine that is seizing up. You feel tired all the time, it is hard to perform everyday chores, everything is an effort, and it seems as if everything is slowed down. Your speech may be slow and monotonous and you may even move slowly. Doctors call this "psychomotor retardation."

Sometimes bodily functions slow down or seize up as well. You may find that you have a dry mouth or that you become constipated; some women stop menstruating or their periods may become irregular.

Loss of appetite

When you are depressed you can lose quite a lot of weight. Food seems unappetizing and bland and you don't even feel hungry. Some people with severe depression stop eating and drinking completely, but this is rare.

Reverse physical symptoms

Instead of the normal physical symptoms of depression such as poor sleep, loss of appetite, and loss of weight, some people have what are known as "reverse physical symptoms." They sleep more, have a bigger appetite, and gain weight. If you feel low in mood and have these symptoms you should see your doctor.

Other physical symptoms

Depression can produce just about any physical symptom. Pain and a feeling of pressure are common, most often affecting the head, face, back, chest, and gut. People frequently come to hospital accident and emergency departments complaining of chest pain and worried that something is wrong with their hearts, when in fact they are suffering from depression. The pain is real but is caused by depression; there is nothing wrong with their hearts.

Sex

Many people go off sex when they are depressed. There are many reasons for this. Some people do not feel able to fulfill a physically loving relationship when they are emotionally numb. Other people feel so negative about themselves that they cannot relax. These psychological problems can lead to physical problems. Men may find it difficult to get an erection and women may find that their vaginas are dry and that intercourse is painful. Many people who are depressed cannot say why it is, but they just don't feel interested in sex.

"Smiling" depression

Not everyone with depression feels low—some people say that they do not feel depressed but go to their doctor with bodily symptoms such as pain, headache, or tiredness that point to depression. Physical examination and investigation do not reveal a physical cause for their illness and the only treatment that works is antidepressant medication. It may be that their subconscious mind is playing tricks on them and does not allow their conscious mind to admit that they feel depressed.

What causes the symptoms?
Chemical deficiencies
Low levels of certain chemicals in the brain may cause the symptoms of depression. To understand the reason, we need to look at how the brain works. The brain consists of billions of nerve cells. It can take hundreds of these nerve cells to perform the smallest action, even to think about doing something. In order for nerve cells to work together they have to communicate with each other and they do this by releasing chemicals called neurotransmitters.

Between the end of one nerve cell and the next there is a small space called the synapse. The first nerve cell communicates with the next by releasing neurotransmitters into the synapse. These neurotransmitters attach to the next nerve cells and so pass on the message.

Studies have shown that three important neurotransmitters, dopamine, serotonin, and noradrenaline, are in short supply in depression. The levels are low in the synapses, and this leads to faulty brain communication and message passing which may be the cause of depressive symptoms.

Nobody knows what causes these low levels of the chemicals. Scientists do not know whether:

- they cause the depressed mood
- they are caused by the depressed mood.

It may be that low levels of neurotransmitters are caused by stress which then leads to depression. Antidepressant drugs work by increasing the levels of these neurotransmitter chemicals.

The role of hormones

Hormones may be important in causing depression. The role of female hormones in depression is discussed on page 103. This section discusses the role of stress hormones. Depression is closely linked to stressful experiences.

Stress hormones

When you are stressed your body releases a complex series of hormones. First, your brain releases the corticotrophin-releasing factor, a hormone that triggers the release of adrenocorticotrophic hormone (ACTH). ACTH travels in the bloodstream to the abdomen where it causes two small glands perched on top of your kidneys (the adrenal glands) to release cortisol.

Cortisol, corticotrophin-releasing factor, and ACTH work together with adrenaline (epinephrine) to make you feel scared and anxious and get your body ready to deal with the source of the stress.

In most people, hormone levels return to normal once the stressful situation has passed but, in depression, the system is hyperactive and cortisol levels do not follow the normal pattern.

In healthy people, cortisol is usually released in large quantities in the morning and in diminishing amounts throughout the day, whereas in some depressed people

How nerve cells transmit signals

Essentially, your brain is like a bundle of telephone wires transmitting and receiving messages within your brain and to and from other parts of your body. Some of the messages are sent by electrical impulses; others depend on the release and transmission of particular chemicals called neurotransmitters.

Nerve cell 1

Axon

Message

Neurotransmitter molecules (dopamine)

Synaptic knob

Message transmission
Neurotransmitter molecules cross the synaptic cleft and attach to the receptor sites, so passing on the message

Vesicles

Synaptic cleft

Nerve cell 2

Receptor sites

Cerebrum

Cerebellum

Brain stem

Spinal cord

its release is the same all day long. Nobody knows whether this leads to depression or is the result of it, but cortisol is known to affect the levels of neurotransmitters in the brain.

Measurement of the changing levels of cortisol in the body has led to a test for depression, but it is not that sensitive and works only in about three of ten people. It works best in those who have serious depression with physical symptoms.

Brain cell death and growth

As our ability to investigate the brain has increased, we have developed better understanding of what is happening in depression.

Stress and depressed mood not only change the levels of hormones and neurotransmitters but also have subtle effects on the structure of the brain. They also temporarily affect the rate of death and birth of nerve cells. During bouts of depression, some small areas of the brain seem to shrink and there are changes in the blood flow. Recent research has demonstrated that some antidepressants protect nerve cells from death, but it is not yet clear how important this is to how effectively they work.

KEY POINTS

- Depression has physical as well as mental symptoms

- Symptoms vary from person to person

- Anyone who thinks about suicide is at risk of committing it and should seek help urgently

Causes of depression

Why me, why now?

The questions most often asked by people who are depressed are "Why me?" and "Why now?"

Sometimes there is an obvious cause for depression, such as bereavement, loss of a job, or physical sickness. But often there is none. To complicate the situation still further, depression doesn't affect everyone who is bereaved, loses their job, or gets sick. We all have strengths and weaknesses. Some people may be more at risk of depression than others but, given the right circumstances, any of us could become depressed.

Researchers have a long way to go before they understand why people become depressed. Often there is more than one cause and having a problem that makes you prone to depression does not mean that you will develop it.

Factors that may make you prone to depression

Genes

Genes (the biological code that you inherit from your parents) are important in depression but there are many genes involved and no one knows exactly how they work. There is certainly no evidence of straightforward inheritance for most forms of depression.

You will not definitely develop depression because your mother, father, sister, or brother has it, but your risk will be increased. You will be at highest risk if you have an identical twin who has developed depression.

It is difficult to place a figure on this risk because the importance of genes is different for different types of depression. They are more important in severe than in mild depression and more important in young people who get depressed than in older people who get depressed. Genes are most important in the minority of people who have periods when their moods are high and periods when their moods are low—this is known as bipolar disorder or manic depression.

Even if there is depression in the family, there will usually need to be some sort of stressful life event to trigger it.

Personality

No single type of personality predisposes people to depression. However, those who are obsessional, dogmatic, and rigid, and who tend to hide their feelings, may be more at risk, as may those who get anxious easily.

People who have repeated and sustained up-and-down moods are more likely to develop manic–depressive illness. However, the vast majority of people who have depression do not have any of these personality types.

Family environment
Losing a parent in childhood
There is some evidence that people who lose their mother when they are young have an increased risk of depression. Suffering that sort of loss might scar you psychologically and make you more susceptible to depression but, on the other hand, it might make you more resilient. It may be the psychological, social, and financial consequences of losing a parent, rather than the loss itself, that are important.

Type of parenting

Psychologists claim that demanding, critical parents who take any success for granted but are harsh on any kind of failure may make their children more prone to depression in the future. Psychotherapists have suggested that people who have little maternal affection when they are young are at risk of depression in later life but there is no scientific proof for this.

Physical or sexual abuse in childhood

There is some evidence that physical or sexual abuse can make people prone to severe depression in later life. Studies have shown that up to half of the people who see a psychiatrist have had some kind of unwanted sexual attention during early adolescence or childhood.

People who have been abused generally remember the abuse but some people first remember childhood abuse when they are depressed and having psychotherapy. There is disagreement between specialists as to whether these memories are always real. Some argue that, on rare occasions, psychotherapists who believe that sexual abuse is the cause of their patient's problem can make the patients remember things that never actually happened by suggesting to them that they did. This is known as "false memory syndrome."

Gender

Women are twice as likely to be diagnosed as being depressed as men. This does not necessarily mean that women are more prone to depression. It may be that women are more likely to admit to depression than men or that doctors are more likely to recognize it in

Factors that influence depression

Both long-standing factors and current difficulties may play a part in causing someone to become depressed.

Factors that may make you prone to depression:

- Genes
- Personality
- Family environment
- Gender
- Thinking patterns
- Having little control over your destiny
- Stress and life events
- Physical illness
- Lack of daylight

Factors that can trigger depression:

- Stress
- Physical illness
- Prescription medication
- Lack of daylight

women. There are, however, social pressures on women that lead to depression that men are less likely to encounter—such as being alone at home with small children. There are also hormonal changes throughout the menstrual cycle and those related to pregnancy, childbirth, and the menopause that may make women more prone to become depressed or to trigger a bout of depressive illness. (For more on this, see page 103.)

Thinking patterns

In 1967, Aaron Beck, an American psychiatrist, described patterns of thinking that are common in depression and that he thought made people prone to getting depression. In short, he believed that people who are very negative about themselves are prone to getting depression.

Most of us have an optimistic way of thinking which keeps us moderately cheerful most of the time. We tend to belittle our failures and make the most of our successes. For example, if you spill a drink in a crowded bar you may say the glasses were overfilled or someone pushed you—it was not your fault. However, if you get through the mass of people without spilling a drop you may be unlikely to say that the glasses were underfilled or everyone else was careful not to push you. You may claim it as a feat of skill.

Some people who are prone to depression think the other way around. They tend to belittle their successes and dwell on their failures. There is evidence that people think like this when they are depressed, but there is no good evidence that they think like this before they get depressed. The importance of this theory is that it has led to "cognitive therapy," one of the most exciting new treatments for depression (see page 65).

Having little control over your destiny

Some specialists believe that people placed for a long time in a situation over which they have no power and from which they cannot escape are prone to develop depression.

The idea came from experiments on dogs performed by a psychologist. He found that they became demoralized and passive, and ate less if they were put in experimental conditions where they were given mild punishment for no apparent reason and consequently had no way of controlling it. He called this "learned helplessness."

Other specialists believe that it is difficult to equate the actions of dogs with those of humans and it is very difficult to say whether dogs ever get depressed. However, rates of depression are high in those bed-bound or wheelchair-bound patients who have to rely on nurses for everything.

Long-term disabling illnesses

Discomfort, disability, dependency, and insecurity can make it more likely that a person will become depressed. Most of us prefer to be independent and like to meet people. Being forced into a position where they are relatively helpless may be one way in which severely ill people become prone to depression or it may be that the energy needed to fight off depression is sapped by long-term illnesses. Worries over financial insecurity may also be important.

Factors that may trigger depression
Stress and life events

Stress can lead to depression whether it comes in the form of a sudden, overwhelming event or as long-term stress. Depression is six times more common in the six months after a markedly stressful life event. Stress can make you more prone to developing depression or can trigger it.

Top 10 stressful life events

- Death of a spouse
- Divorce
- Marital separation
- Prison term
- Death of a close friend
- Injury or illness
- Marriage
- Losing your job
- Marital reconciliation
- Retirement

Life events such as loss of a partner or loss of a job may be the final straw if you have long-term difficulties such as housing, marriage, and/or work problems. The long-term problems magnify the effect of the short-term problem.

The experiences that trigger depression are usually losses of some kind—such as losing your job, the death of someone you love (see Grief and Bereavement, page 121), or the loss of a partner through divorce. However, there may also be losses of a more subtle kind, such as loss of self-esteem through a destructive relationship.

Only one in ten of such "loss events" leads to depression, and other experiences in life that sometimes trigger depression do not involve loss of any kind. We all have our own psychological ways of reacting to stress and it is not possible to predict how we will react.

Some illnesses linked with depression

- Acromegaly
- Addison's disease
- Alcohol: direct effect on the brain and also because it ruins your life
- Brain abscess
- Brain hemorrhage
- Brain tumors
- Chronic fatigue syndrome
- Cushing's disease
- Dementia
- Diabetes
- Encephalitis
- Head injuries
- Heart problems
- Hyperparathyroidism
- Hypopituitarism
- Hypothyroidism
- Multiple sclerosis
- Parkinson's disease
- Severe head injury
- Tuberculosis, meningitis
- Vitamin deficiency
- Viral illnesses (including flu and glandular fever (infectious mononucleosis))
- Water balance problems (such as low salt, high calcium, or low calcium in your body)

Physical illness

Physical illness can set off depression. The shock of finding out that you have a serious illness can lead to a loss of confidence and self-esteem, and so to depression. But the reasons are complex: for instance, depression is quite common after a heart attack, possibly because people feel that they had a near miss and it makes them face their own mortality, or perhaps because they become suddenly disabled. In older people, physical illness is one of the most common causes of depression.

Some illnesses can cause depression because of the way that they affect the body. Depression can accompany Parkinson's disease and multiple sclerosis partly because of their effects on the brain. Illnesses that affect the hormones can cause depression.

There's also a link with viral illnesses: an epidemic of influenza is often followed by an epidemic of depression and many of us will know someone who has become depressed after a bout of glandular fever (infectious mononucleosis). How a virus causes depression is not clear, but one theory is that viruses use up the body's supplies of vitamins, so weakening it.

Prescription medicines

Some prescription medications can cause depression (see box), but you shouldn't stop taking any of the medicines on the list without consulting your doctor. These drugs do not always cause depression and it may be that you have another

Some medicines that may cause depression

- Anti-epilepsy tablets
- Anti-high blood pressure drugs
- Anti-malarial drug—mefloquine (Lariam)
- Anti-parkinsonian drugs
- Chemotherapy drugs (some) used in the treatment of cancer
- Contraceptive pill (combined contraceptive pill and possibly the progestogen-only pill)
- Digitalis (heart)
- Diuretics (heart and blood pressure)
- Interferon-alfa used in the treatment of hepatitis C
- Major tranquilizers
- Steroid therapy (for asthma, arthritis, etc.)

reason for being depressed. Sometimes stopping the medication that you are taking can be more dangerous than the depression.

Non-prescription medication can also lead to depression. Alcohol has direct effects on the brain and can make you feel depressed. Alcoholism can also cause depression because of the negative effect that it has on your life. Similarly recreational drugs can have an effect through direct effects and the impact that they have on your lifestyle.

Lack of daylight
Most of us feel better in the sun than on overcast days and prefer the summer to the winter, but this takes an

extreme form in some individuals. They are fine in summer but become depressed as the days grow shorter at the onset of winter. They are said to suffer from "seasonal affective disorder (SAD)."

SAD may be related to the levels of a hormone called melatonin which is released from the pineal gland in the brain. Its release is sensitive to light; more is released when it is dark. Light therapy is sometimes very effective in getting rid of the symptoms of seasonal affective disorder. Four hours of bright light a day from a special lamp can lift depression within a week.

KEY POINTS

- There are many possible reasons for depression

- Some physical illnesses and some medications cause depression

- Usually there are a number of causes for any person's depressive illness

Types of depression

Classifying depression

When you see a doctor, counselor, or other professional, you may hear a variety of terms used to describe your illness. Some have overlapping meanings, but in this book the terms mild, moderate, and severe are used throughout to describe depression, and these have clear distinguishing characteristics.

Mild depression

In mild depression, the low mood may come and go and the illness often starts after a specific stressful event. The person may feel anxious as well as feeling low. Lifestyle changes are often all that are needed to lift this kind of depression.

Moderate depression

In moderate depression, low mood is persistent and the person has physical symptoms as well, although they will vary from person to person. Changes in lifestyle alone are unlikely to work and medical help is needed.

Severe depression

Severe depression is a life-threatening illness in which the symptoms are intense. The person will experience physical symptoms, delusions, and hallucinations, and it is important to see a doctor as soon as possible.

Other terms for depression

Other terms in common use in the medical profession to describe types of depression include the following.

Reactive depression

This term is used in two ways by doctors. In the first, reactive is used to describe a depression that is caused by a stressful event—such as losing your job—and doesn't usually last long. It could be described as a short-lived exaggeration of a normal response to adversity. Counseling, family support, stress management, and practical steps may be all that are needed to treat it.

However, a stressful event can trigger more severe depression and people who are prone to depression can have stressful life events after their illness starts. If this happens it is difficult to pinpoint exactly whether the depression is truly a reaction to stress.

The term "reactive" is also used to describe a depression in which a person can still react to and enjoy social situations.

Endogenous depression

Endogenous depression comes on for no reason; it is usually intense and the person is likely to have physical symptoms such as loss of appetite and weight, early morning wakening, mood worse in the morning, and loss of interest in sex. It will usually improve only with treatment.

The trouble with using this particular way of defining depression is that the same symptoms can be triggered in some people by stressful events. Also, just because you can't put your finger on any particular stressful event that set the depression off, it doesn't mean that there wasn't one.

Neurotic depression

This term is used to describe a mild form of depression in which the person has good and bad days. They tend to feel more depressed in the evenings. With this kind of depression, you may well experience difficulty getting to sleep and have interrupted sleep but no early morning wakening. Some people sleep excessively and some find that they are more irritable than usual. Neurotic can be used as a term of abuse so the description "neurotic depression" is not used much these days and, in any case, it is really just another name for mild depression.

Psychotic depression

Psychotic depression is severe and people who have it will experience physical symptoms and may lose touch with reality. They may have delusions and/or hallucinations. People with psychotic depression always need medical treatment.

Bipolar disorder

Bipolar disorder or depression is another name for manic–depressive illness. People with manic–depressive illness have sustained high moods and periods of sustained low moods that can range from mild to severe depression.

When people with this illness are in one of the high moods (manic), they are likely to feel elated, need less sleep or food than usual, and experience a general feeling of well-being. They have excessive amounts of energy, speak very quickly, and feel as if thoughts are racing in their head. Their judgment is likely to be poor and they may also experience delusions and hallucinations but these are the opposite to those in depression—their content is much more positive. Some people believe that they know celebrities or are VIPs when they are not, others that they are very wealthy or have special powers. High moods can be even more destructive than low ones and sometimes the lack of sound judgment and delusions can lead to financial trouble as a result of impulse buying—perhaps on a credit card spree.

Unipolar depression
Unipolar depression is a term that is used to describe the kind of depression experienced by the vast majority of people and means that they have only low moods, not high ones as well.

Agitated depression
Agitated depression is actually a description of the symptoms of this type of depression, in which the individual is anxious, worried, and restless.

Retarded depression
Retarded depression is again a description of symptoms and refers to the kind of depression in which both mental

and physical processes are slowed down and the person often finds it difficult to concentrate. When the illness is very severe, some people find it impossible to move, speak, or eat and there is a risk that they could starve.

Dysthymia
This terms refers to mild depression that is persistent. Although it may come and go, doctors will make this diagnosis if the illness has lasted for more than two months in two years. The main symptoms are indecision and low self-esteem. Psychotherapy may work better than drug treatment.

Masked (smiling) depression
People with masked depression say they do not feel depressed even though they have a number of other symptoms that point to depression. They may be investigated for physical illnesses before the diagnosis is made. Symptoms such as chest pain or sleep problems diminish when the person is given antidepressant treatment.

Organic depression
This is the name given to a kind of depression that is caused by a physical illness or medication.

Brief recurrent depression
This is a recently recognized illness in which serious depression comes on but lasts for only a few days at a time.

Seasonal affective disorder (SAD)
This term was originally used to mean any depressive illness that came on regularly at a certain time of year—

say because of increased demands at work. It is now used for a specific type of depression that may result from decreasing levels of daylight as winter approaches and days get shorter. People with SAD may experience cravings for carbohydrates and/or chocolate, and an increased need for sleep.

KEY POINTS

- There are many types of depression

- Mild depression may not need drug treatment, but moderate and severe depression often do

- Depression may be constant or intermittant

- Depression may be associated with symptoms other than mood

Helping yourself

Involve your doctor

Many people with mild depression get better by using simple self-help measures alone. There are lots of examples of guided self-help plans that you can get from your primary care physician or even on the Internet.

Even if you decide that you are going to use self-help alone, it is still worth seeing your doctor for a number of reasons. For instance your depression may be caused by a physical illness. Also, if your doctor assesses you again at a later date, he or she will be in a position to give you an independent view as to whether self-help has worked for you.

People with more severe forms of depression will also benefit from self-help measures, but they should be used as part of a plan discussed with the doctor and a psychiatrist or other therapist. Self-help measures may help stave off depression as well as treat it and promote recovery. Do not try to do everything at once—consider which of the suggestions could make a difference to you and then try one. You will feel better for it.

Be prepared for difficulties

People often become depressed following a loss of some kind, but sometimes it may be possible to prepare yourself when you know you are going to have to face up to a change. The kind of predictable situations that can trigger depression include loss of family support when a person goes to college, loss of freedom or work status when a woman takes maternity leave, and loss of work routine and social contact for some people when they retire. Not surprisingly, rates of depression are high at around these times.

There are two ways to decrease the stress of predictable loss:

(1) being open and acknowledging that there may be a problem

(2) by preparing for the change.

If you acknowledge your feelings you will feel better. If you are worried about the change in your life, talk it through with a friend—let other people know your concerns and they may be able to support you. Saying how you feel may change the way they treat you: for example, if you are retiring, they may stop telling you that you should be glad not to have to work any more, they may spend more time with you or expect less of you while you're adjusting to your new situation.

Good preparation for any change is helpful; reading about it, or talking to people who have gone through a similar experience will be useful. Taking commonsense measures to decrease the stress and trying to arrange your first few days or weeks in advance may help the transition.

For instance, if you are going to college, you may find that there are people you know there whom you could arrange to meet up with or you could practice cooking some simple meals before you go so you have one less problem to worry about. The early weeks of retirement can be planned so that there is social support and you have something to do. Many women find support groups invaluable after they have had a baby.

Take a break
If you are feeling blue or you feel that everything is getting on top of you, take a break, even if you can manage only a day or a night away. Better still, take a proper vacation if you can. It is not running away from

your problems and you will get only a little behind in your work. You will probably find that you may be able to think things through better if you are away from them and you may work better when you get back. A break may give you the rest you need to attack your problems and the distance to put them in proper perspective. If you find you cannot enjoy a few days away, this is a sign that you need professional help.

Talk things over

You will find that, if you talk problems over with your partner, a friend, or family member, you will feel better. It not only decreases the burden on you, but just talking through things may also help you find a solution.

You may discover that your friends have their own ideas about what you should do and may think of solutions that haven't occurred to you. They may have gone through the same kind of difficulties that you are experiencing and so be able to give you insights into your problems.

People often feel better after they have had a good cry. The open acknowledgment of your problems is often the starting point for working out solutions.

Many people who are depressed cut themselves off and think that they are a burden to other people. In fact, this just makes you more depressed so try instead to choose a friend who will be sympathetic and willing to listen to you and help you through a difficult time. Everyone needs help at some time.

Change your lifestyle

See whether you can identify and change aspects of your life that may have brought on the depression. You may need help to do this but it is not as impractical as it seems. Somebody else has usually gone through the same problem before and there may be a way in which you can solve it too. If you are worried about an illness you should discuss this with your doctor; things may not be as bad as they seem. If it is a social or legal problem you could visit a legal advice center for help.

Get in touch with a group

There are many ways in which other people can help and joining a group of some kind can be a real support. Some possibilities that you might consider are listed in the section starting on page 133. The local department of psychiatry will also have information about what is available in your area. You can also call a hotline number, nationwide or in your state, to get confidential advice. There are a number of other organizations that offer more specialized help—for example helping with relationship difficulties, drug and alcohol problems or domestic violence. See the "Useful information" section on page 133.

Exercise

Exercise can boost your well-being too. It doesn't just make you feel better psychologically; it also gets you out of the house and makes you fitter. It does not have to be strenuous aerobics. Going for a good walk or a swim will do just as well. Active pastimes, such as bowling, are a good way of getting out and doing something. If you have not done any exercise for a while, you should be careful and start slowly.

When you are feeling low, it is sometimes hard to be motivated to exercise. Getting involved in a structured and supervised exercise program can be the best way to make sure that you do enough but not too much, and that you continue to do it. Your doctor can often offer advice on this.

Can you eat yourself happy?

The importance of a balanced diet
Diet is an important element in keeping depression at bay. Although it is unlikely that you will be able to eat yourself happy, it is important to eat properly during a bout of depression and a regular balanced diet with all the essential vitamins that may keep you feeling well when the bout is over.

If you are suffering from depression, cutting out caffeine is a good idea because it can make you feel anxious, and eating large amounts of carbohydrates may produce mood swings and so is best avoided.

What you eat may be more important in staving off depression than treating it when you are already feeling low.

Food that may improve your mood
Selenium (oysters, mushrooms, Brazil nuts), zinc (shellfish, seafood, eggs), and chromium (green vegetables, poultry—especially turkey and dietary supplements from health food stores) have been suggested as nutrients that might improve your mood, but they should not be taken in high doses. A qualified nutritionist can give you more advice on healthy eating.

Some scientists claim that eating fish can help depression. This is because studies have shown that fish oils have antidepressant and mood-stabilizing properties. Unfortunately, you would have to eat an awful lot of fish to get enough fish oil to make any difference. As a result, some companies have started to produce capsules that contain concentrated fish oil. Most people have no side effects, though they

Can you eat yourself happy? (contd)

may get a slightly upset stomach. Unfortunately, their impact on mood is far from proven.

Eating a balanced diet rich in mood-enhancing foods and cutting out too much carbohydrate, caffeine, and alcohol is generally good for you, whether or not it cures a bout of depression.

If you think you may be deficient in essential nutrients such as vitamins and minerals you should talk this over with your doctor who can refer you to a nutritionist.

Look after yourself
Activities

If you are feeling depressed, keeping occupied often helps. Try taking up a new activity or hobby at an evening class or at the weekend. Getting out of the house and meeting people will do you good because it breaks the vicious circle of loneliness and spending too much time mulling over your problems.

Make a conscious effort to do what you like doing best. It may be listening to a CD, shopping, having a massage, going to a concert or a movie. Little things can make a big difference.

Food and nutrition

Even if you do not have much of an appetite, make sure that you eat regularly and, if you cannot face a meal, go for balanced snacks instead. If you do not eat correctly, you will not have the physical strength to recover and you will start descending into the vicious circle of worse and worse depression. If you really cannot face eating properly, or preparing a meal, meal substitutes, such as Ensure, can be bought from pharmacies without a prescription. They contain a whole day's nourishment in liquid form and are easy to prepare.

Alcohol

Remember that alcohol will not solve your problems. It will make you feel more depressed and could become a habit that ruins your life. Alcohol decreases inhibitions and may lead to suicidal impulses taking over. You should also be careful about drinking alcohol if you are taking antidepressants. Always check with your doctor if you are on medication and intend to drink alcohol.

Alcohol will not sort out your problems.

Sleep

Sleeping problems are common in depressed people who are especially prone to insomnia. Lack of sleep makes it more difficult to summon up the energy to fight depression.

If your depression is moderate or severe, self-help may not be enough and you may need medication to sort out your insomnia.

Stress management

Relaxation

This is easier said than done and is something that we all need help with but there are many ways of relieving tension and one of them will work for you. One thing that many relaxation techniques have in common is that they teach you to recognize when your muscles are tense and how to relieve the tension. You can learn this by going to a relaxation group, buying relaxation tapes, or by reading about relaxation. This is often a good place to start and after a couple of sessions you will probably be able to do it by yourself.

There are more elaborate methods of relaxation such as meditation and yoga, and fancy sounding ways of teaching you to know when you are tense such as biofeedback.

Biofeedback relaxation

This is aided by a machine that monitors either muscle responses or electrical activity in the skin. When you are more tense, electrical activity in the skin and muscle increases and this causes the machine to produce a signal—either a high-pitched whistle or a light coming on. When you relax the sound gets lower in frequency

How to get a good night's sleep

Prolonged bouts of insomnia can be very stressful and will make your depression much more difficult to cope with. Listed below are some useful tips to help you get a good night's sleep.

- Get up earlier in the morning to see if this helps
- Take some exercise during the day
- Do not take naps
- Do not exercise just before bed—it can make it difficult to sleep
- Do not have a heavy meal late at night; you could feel uncomfortable—but do not go to bed hungry
- Do not drink coffee, tea, or sodas in the evening
- Have a milky warm drink last thing before going to bed
- Get your mind off your problems by reading a book before trying to sleep
- Go to bed at a regular time so that your body sets up a natural rhythm
- Do not drink alcohol to help you sleep—it may not work and you may not be able to break the habit
- Make sure your bed is comfortable
- Make sure the room is not too hot or too cold
- Try to stop smoking. If you smoke, do not smoke before you go to sleep—nicotine is a stimulant and there is a danger of fire
- Sexual intercourse before you go to sleep can help you wind down

How to get a good night's sleep (contd)

- Perform relaxation exercises before you go to bed
- Remember—if you can't get off to sleep for half an hour, or if you wake up at night and can't get back to sleep, get up and read a little, drink some hot milk, and then try to go back to sleep. Lying there worrying will not do you any good—it could make things worse!

or the light goes out—so you learn how to relax your muscles.

Autogenic training
This is a series of simple mental exercises in which the patient is encouraged to enter a state of passive concentration—it is a form of meditation that can reduce stress and make people more relaxed.

You will usually need professional help for these exercises, and many of the techniques involved in autogenic training are no more effective than simple relaxation training.

Massage
This can be done by yourself, your partner, or a professional. There are plenty of devices that can be bought to help you massage yourself, but it is usually best to get someone else to do it. You may be able to talk over your problems at the same time. Specialist types of massage, Shiatsu, reflexology, and aromatherapy, are all good for stress.

Relaxation exercise

This is a simple method for relaxing. It only takes 20 minutes maximum. You can do it in bed, lying on the floor, or sitting in a comfortable chair. Just make sure that any chair you use supports your neck. You may want to try it in the evening first time around—some people feel so relaxed that they fall asleep. Once you've got the hang of it you will be able to do it anywhere without dropping off, unless you want to.

1. Let your whole body go limp. Try to feel as heavy on the bed or in the chair as possible. Let the bed or the chair take your weight. Feel heavy, like a sack of potatoes.

2. Put your arms by your side and let them flop down. Let your legs go all floppy as well. Let your shoulders drop. Relax all parts of your body from the top down. Feel heavy on the bed or chair.

3. If you have not performed relaxation exercises before, you will need to teach yourself how to relax your muscles. Tense the muscle in your upper leg harder and harder until you can't do it any more. Now release it. You will feel the

Relaxation exercise (contd)

difference between tension and relaxation. Do the same from the top of your body to your toes. Start with your face—screw your face up, clench your teeth, and then release. Then make your neck muscles tense, then release. Shrug your shoulders so that they nearly touch your ears, then let them drop. Tense and release your arms, chest, stomach, butt, legs, feet, and toes, one by one.

4. You will find that your muscles feel less tense than they did when you started. Remember what they feel like. Once you have the hang of it you will not need to tense your muscles before you relax them.

5. When you feel relaxed and limp, slow your breathing down bit by bit, making it slow and even. Concentrate only on your breathing. Make inhaling and exhaling the same length, long and slow. Stop if you feel light-headed. After 20 minutes, you will feel much better than when you started. You will feel much calmer and more rested.

Shiatsu
This is a Japanese massage technique built on traditional Chinese medical theory. Our vital life force or Qi is believed to flow through our bodies in certain pathways or meridians. If it gets blocked or there is an imbalance it leads to disease. In Shiatsu massage, pressure points are manipulated to unblock or balance Qi.

Reflexology
This is another ancient art of massage. Different areas on the foot are thought to be linked to certain body systems. Manipulation and massage of these areas are thought to put right problems that you have in the particular body system.

Aromatherapy
This uses the scents of plant oils and essential oils to aid psychological well-being.

Pet therapy
Some people who are prone to recurrent depression find that it is therapeutic to get a dog or a cat. They are cuddly, reliable, and responsive and may decrease your stress level. However, being given a pet when you are depressed will not necessarily make you feel better. Apart from the fact that a pet requires a lot of time and effort, it takes time to build up a relationship.

Complementary medicine
Homeopathy
Homeopathy is a form of medicine built on the principle that like heals like but that very small quantities of a substance can promote healing. There is little research to support this but many people claim to

benefit from such treatment. These treatments are not usually considered dangerous but before going to see a homoeopath of your own accord, it is wise to talk it over with your doctor first.

Acupuncture

Acupuncture works on the same principles of Qi as Shiatsu; however, fine needles are inserted to points on the meridians to help balance Qi rather than massage. This is increasingly being used in the relief of pain and anxiety. There are a number of doctors who are trained in acupuncture as well as in conventional western medicine. Its use in depression is still a matter for debate.

Chinese herbal medicine

Chinese herbalists have been treating common problems, such as depression, for centuries. It is unclear how effective their remedies are. If you decide to see one or take a prescription, make sure that you tell your primary care physician or psychiatrist. Some herbal cures interact with other drugs that your doctor may give you.

Hypnosis

This can be used to aid relaxation but is not a treatment for depression. In hypnosis you enter a trance, you are not asleep, and the hypnotist attempts to help you manipulate your subconscious mind. Some types of hypnosis have been used to stop people feeling anxious but there is little evidence for them working to cure depression.

KEY POINTS

- Self-help can be used as part of a plan agreed with your doctor

- Do not try to change everything all at one time

- Once you are well, self-help techniques may stave off depression in the future

Treatment

Talking to your doctor

If self-help does not work, or if your depression is severe from the outset you should see your primary care physician or a psychiatrist. He or she:

- is knowledgeable about depression
- will listen to you
- may know you and know your medical history

- can make sure that there are no physical problems that are causing the depression
- can arrange investigations or start treatment
- will be there to offer you support
- can sign you off work sick if need be
- can refer you to a psychiatrist if your health care coverage does not allow for self-referral
- will know of other therapies available in your area.

If there is an emergency, such as feeling suicidal, you should call your doctor immediately or go straight to your local emergency room. There, you will be assessed by a doctor and a psychiatrist can be called if necessary. In some areas hospitals have emergency, walk-in psychiatric clinics.

In all of these services the professionals are used to dealing with people who are depressed and will offer high-quality treatment. No one will think that your problems are trivial or stupid. They will be eager to help—that is what they are there for.

Types of treatment
There are three types of treatment for depression:

(1) psychological treatments

(2) drug treatment (see page 70)

(3) physical treatments (see page 93).

Psychological treatments are dealt with in this chapter and medication and physical treatments in the next two.

Psychotherapy—talking therapies
Psychotherapy, or "talk therapy," is a popular type of treatment for depression, partly because it does not

involve taking tablets and partly because it makes intuitive sense. It seems right to sit down and talk about things if they are getting on top of us. It also seems right to try to get to the bottom of why we feel the way we do when depression comes on for no reason.

However, you may be too depressed to be able to think clearly and may be too tired to start psychotherapy. All psychological therapies take a lot of time and commitment. They are not an easy option. They take a lot of energy. If your depression is severe, you may need to lift your depression with antidepressant medication before you consider psychological treatment. You should see your doctor to discuss what is available in your area.

There are many different types of psychological therapy and they are based on different theories. They are most easily split into:

● brief therapies that last at most six months

Treating different types of depression

Depending on whether your psychiatrist or another therapist judges your depression to be mild, moderate, or severe, different kinds of treatment will be recommended.

Mild depression
Self-help, lifestyle changes, and psychotherapy often work. Medication will often be prescribed only if self-help, exercise, and forms of psychotherapy have not worked. Medication is not as effective in mild depression and the side effects can outweigh the beneficial effects.

Moderate depression
Either medication or specific forms of psychotherapy can work here, depending on your symptoms. Some doctors believe that a combination of both is required. If you have early morning wakening, depression worse in the morning, loss of appetite or weight, and loss of interest in things that you used to enjoy, antidepressants will work and work well. However, cognitive, behavioral, and interpersonal therapy also work well in moderate depression and, if they are available and you would prefer not to take medication, you could try these types of therapy first. See your doctor regularly so that you can be monitored. If things get worse you should reconsider starting medication.

- long-term therapies that last longer
- counseling.

Brief therapies usually consist of 4 to 20 weekly sessions, each lasting up to an hour. In long-term therapies, there

Treating different types of depression (contd)

Severe depression

Many people with severe depression are too ill to benefit from psychotherapy and need to start taking antidepressants. People who are actively suicidal need urgent help and to be in a safe place.

If the depression is characterized by delusions and hallucinations, an antidepressant may need to be combined with a special drug, an anti-psychotic, that will specifically treat these symptoms.

Recurrent depression

If you have been depressed before you should use the treatment that worked last time because it will do so again. Once you are well you should discuss long-term treatment with your doctor—lithium or a low dose of antidepressant can help stave off another attack.

Bipolar disorder or manic–depressive illness

Depression can be treated with antidepressants but your doctor will want to monitor your treatment carefully because, in a few people with up-and-down moods, antidepressants can lead to a high mood. In the long term, other medications that act as mood stabilizers—such as lithium—may be more suitable.

are usually over 50 sessions; they are often weekly but they can be as frequently as five times a week. Brief therapies usually deal with problems in the here-and-now, whereas long-term therapies delve into the past to try to discover why you are the way that you are.

Counseling lasts for a variable time, from a single session onward. It does not aim to change deep-rooted problems or treat your depression, but it may help get rid of some of the problems that are causing you to be depressed.

Brief therapies

Many brief therapies are available and your psychiatrist may suggest that you try one of these. The possibilities include:

- cognitive therapy
- cognitive analytical therapy
- cognitive–behavioral therapy
- behavioral therapy
- interpersonal therapy.

All of these have been used in depression.

The kind of therapy you are offered may depend on what is available locally. Getting a good therapist is important, but the type of therapy that you get is also important. Many specialists currently favor cognitive–behavioral therapy and interpersonal therapy (see pages 66 and 67) over other brief therapies. Studies suggest that they can be as good as antidepressant treatment for treating bouts of moderate depression and decrease the risk of a relapse. Your therapist may be a doctor, a nurse, a psychologist, or a social worker.

There has been little guidance on how long a course of brief therapy should last. However, many of the studies that show benefit in depression use 16 to 20 sessions of therapy over a 6- to 9-month period.

Following this, some also offer two to four top-up sessions over the following six to 12 months.

Cognitive therapy

Cognitive therapy works specifically on depressive thinking patterns. You will be asked to record your negative thoughts and look at the way that you think. You will then be helped to challenge thoughts that are unrealistically negative. Over 10 to 20 weekly sessions, the therapist tries to help you to stop thinking in a depressed way. This has been shown to work in even moderately severe depression. It can have benefits that last longer than medication alone and can be used in combination with antidepressants. You should consider it seriously.

For instance, our secretary Carrie from page 10 would be asked to work through her belief that she is a failure and present evidence for and against it. She would be helped to see that there are other ways of looking at the problem and that she does not have to be so hard on herself. She would be helped to think in a more balanced way. Perhaps she is not the best secretary in the world but she is a good secretary and even good secretaries make mistakes from time to time.

Behavioral therapy

This differs from cognitive therapy in that it focuses on what we do rather than what we think. Rather than trying to make you *think* less depressed, it makes you *act* less depressed. A behavior modification program may attempt to get you sleeping well, looking after yourself better, and eating better. It stops you "giving up." Some people find this an effective first step to recovery.

In Carrie's case, all of these may be employed to make sure that she does not slip into more severe depression. She would be encouraged to look after herself, have good sleeping and eating habits, and make sure that she does not get into a depressive downward spiral.

Cognitive–behavioral therapy

This combines elements of cognitive therapy and behavioral therapy. It can be a potent treatment of mild and moderate depression. Trials have shown that it can be as effective as antidepressant drugs. It has been shown to get you better and keep you better. It can be used alone, but some studies have shown that the combination of cognitive–behavioral therapy and antidepressants is better than either one alone.

Cognitive analytical therapy

This is another new therapy. It uses cognitive and behavioral techniques but also looks into your past to give you an idea about where your ways of thinking come from. It is one of the few brief therapies that looks into the past and gives reasons for your problems.

If Carrie talked about her past it may have become clear that her parents were very critical. Her feelings of inferiority may have come from the way that she was undermined as a child. If she realized that the way she felt was because of circumstances and her childhood, she may find it easier to accept herself for what she is and be less self-critical, dissatisfied, and depressed.

Interpersonal therapy

Interpersonal therapy focuses on people's relationships and on problems such as difficulties in communication or coping with bereavement. Some consider it as effective as cognitive–behavioral therapy. An adequate course of interpersonal therapy is 16 to 20 sessions over a 6-month period.

Computerized therapies

A number of psychological therapies have been computerized, for instance, it is possible to receive cognitive–behavioral therapy via a computer program rather than a therapist. Perhaps surprisingly to some, there are some reports that computerized cognitive–behavioral therapy is effective but more research is needed before it is accepted and widely available.

Long-term therapy

There are many different types of long-term therapy, all based on different theories. Long-term therapies try to deal with the deep-rooted causes of depression. They are not a quick treatment. Their aim is to sort out long-standing problems and they may not make you feel any less depressed in the short term.

Psychoanalysis

Psychoanalysts believe that our difficulties are caused by problems from the past that we have not dealt with. We may have denied them, ignored them, or tried to forget them, but they are still in the back of our minds. They stay there and fester and come back to us when we are under stress or weakened in some way. They can also weaken us. Such a problem could be the loss of a parent or parents when young at which time there was no proper grieving process and feelings were just covered up.

Long-term psychotherapy is said to work by helping these bad feelings come to the surface and into the consciousness. The aim is to disarm them and to stop them causing problems.

If you are considering this type of therapy, you should discuss it with your friends and your doctor or psychiatrist. There is a bewildering choice of psychotherapists and it is always better to get a personal referral or contact a reputable clinic or hospital for a suggested list of practitioners. A reputable therapist will have professional qualifications which they will be happy to explain to you and these can be verified with the relevant state licensing body.

Counseling

Counselors generally try to help you solve problems and may have particular area of experience. They will not usually give specific advice but will help you make decisions. Again, it is a good idea to get a recommendation and enquire into the training the counselor has received prior to commencing treatment.

Couples therapy

Couples therapy is sometimes considered for those who are depressed, have a regular partner, and who have benefited from brief individual therapy. There are many different types of couples therapy. They help couples to discuss their feelings and problems, to work out whether there is anything that they can do as a couple to improve the depression, and to increase both partners' understanding of what is happening. Couples therapy may last for 10 to 20 sessions over a six-month period.

KEY POINTS

- Your primary care physician or psychiatrist should be the first port of call when you need help

- Some brief talking therapies have been shown to work well in depression

- Long-term psychotherapy tries to sort out problems that underlie the depression; it may not lift your depression in the short term

Medication

What is antidepressant medication?

Antidepressant tablets can be a very effective treatment for depression. When they are taken as prescribed and the recommended dosage is given, they often start to improve symptoms in two weeks, though it may take six weeks or more for the full benefit to be felt. You normally continue taking them for at least six months after the depression has vanished to make sure that it does not return, and then gradually stop.

Many doctors aim for someone who has had only one bout of depression to stay on medication for one year and for people who have had many episodes to stay on the medication for at least two years. Some recommend longer periods on antidepressants for older people. They work best for moderate and severe depression.

Will I become addicted?

Many people think they will become addicted to or dependent on antidepressants but this will not happen. Antidepressants are not like Valium (diazepam) and are not addictive. They work only if you are depressed and will not work if you are not. They do not give you a high. There is a black market trade in nearly all drugs that give you a high and can be addictive—there is no black market trade in antidepressants.

However, antidepressants are powerful drugs and some people who stop them suddenly feel weird. This is not a sign that you are dependent on or addicted to antidepressants; people who are addicted crave the drug to which they are addicted; people do not crave antidepressants, it is just that the body is used to having them around. Once you have recovered from depression, a gradual reduction in dose in the weeks before stopping will ensure that your body resets itself and that there are no symptoms.

How do antidepressants work?

In depression, there are physical changes to the way in which your body works and antidepressants can put things back to normal. As we saw earlier (page 18), nerve cells in the brain are separated by a small space —the synapse. In order to pass messages to each other, nerve cells release chemicals (neurotransmitters) which leave one nerve cell and cross the space to the next nerve cell—like a baton in a relay race. The message is passed on only if there is enough neurotransmitter in the synapse. After release the neurotransmitters are broken up or taken back into the brain cell that released them.

The levels of these neurotransmitters are low in depression—it's as if the baton were being dropped. Antidepressants are thought to work by increasing the amount of neurotransmitters in the space between the cells—they put the baton back into the hand of the nerve cell.

The amount of neurotransmitter in the synapse can be increased by various drugs that work in different ways:

- Increasing the amount of neurotransmitter made (L-tryptophan is a chemical found in the diet which is turned into serotonin. It is thought to work by increasing the amount of neurotransmitter made in the brain cells. While available in some countries it is no longer FDA-approved in the United States following a serious side effect connected with L-tryptophan in the 1980s).
- Preventing neurotransmitters being broken down (monoamine oxidase inhibitors or MAOIs).
- Stopping neurotransmitters in the synapse being taken back up into the cells (tricyclics, SSRIs, tricyclic-like compounds).

Over time, the body rights itself, the amounts of neurotransmitters naturally produced increase, and antidepressants are no longer needed.

Who needs antidepressants?

If you are diagnosed with mild depression, you may not need this kind of treatment; with moderate depression you probably do and, with severe depression, you definitely do. In any case, you doctor will help you make this decision.

Medication should be prescribed after a full consultation with a psychiatrist as part of an agreed plan that might also include self-help techniques and psychotherapy. If you are having drug treatment this should be discussed with your therapist. If you are hesitant about taking antidepressants, it might help to remember that doctors do not prescribe antidepressants as an easy alternative to working through your problems. However, you may find it impossible to work through your problems unless you take them.

Certain symptoms—early morning wakening, depression that is worse in the morning, loss of appetite and weight, and loss of interest in things that you used to enjoy—indicate that your depression is very likely to respond to antidepressants.

The medication may have side effects. These are often at their worst when you start treatment but may improve as your body gets used to the drug. They can be reduced by starting at a low dose and building up or changing the drug that you are on. Most side effects are less of a bother than the depression. Again, it may help to remember that the evidence is that if the drugs are taken correctly your depression is very likely to improve.

Antidepressants usually work best if you take a full dose. Low doses may not be as effective and you may end up with side effects but no benefit. Discuss all side effects with your doctor who will help you decide if a change is needed or if you should try to persevere.

Many different antidepressants are available. There is research evidence to show that they all work. Some are better for one type of depression than another and different kinds have different side effects.

After one episode of depression you will be advised to stay on medication for six months to make sure that the depression does not return. If you have had a previous bout of depression you may be advised to stay on medication for longer. Some doctors now advise their patients to stay on medication indefinitely if the depression is severe and there is a significant risk of a

How antidepressants are thought to treat depression

In depression, the levels of neurotransmitters are low.
Antidepressant drugs work to increase levels in one of three ways.

Depressed state (before treatment)

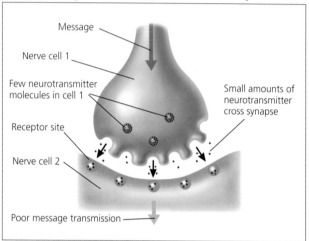

Message

Nerve cell 1

Few neurotransmitter molecules in cell 1

Small amounts of neurotransmitter cross synapse

Receptor site

Nerve cell 2

Poor message transmission

1. Increasing amount of neurotransmitter

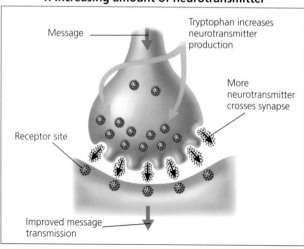

Message

Tryptophan increases neurotransmitter production

More neurotransmitter crosses synapse

Receptor site

Improved message transmission

How antidepressants are thought to treat depression (contd)

2. Stopping breakdown of neurotransmitter

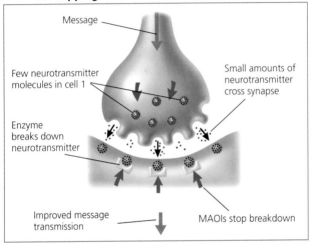

Message

Few neurotransmitter molecules in cell 1

Small amounts of neurotransmitter cross synapse

Enzyme breaks down neurotransmitter

Improved message transmission

MAOIs stop breakdown

3. Inhibiting reabsorption of neurotransmitter

Message

Tricyclics and SSRIs prevent reabsorption of neurotransmitter so more crosses synapse

Few neurotransmitter molecules in cell 1

Enzyme breaks down neurotransmitter

Increased amounts of neurotransmitter cross synapse

Improved message transmission

Examples of Tricyclic antidepressant

The commonly used, or trade names are given first with the generic, or scientific name in parentheses

Sedative tricyclics:

- Elavil (amitriptyline)
- Anafranil (clomipramine)
- Sinequan (doxepin)
- Surmontil (trimipramine)

Stimulant tricyclic:

- Vivactil (protriptyline)

Non-sedative tricyclics:

- Asendin (amoxapine)
- Norpramin (desipramine)
- Tofranil (imipramine)
- Pamelor (nortriptyline)

further bout but this is an individual decision that must be made between you and your doctor.

Different types of antidepressants
Tricyclic antidepressants

These chemicals are called tricyclics because of their chemical structure—three rings that are linked together, with a side chain (like a tricycle). They increase the amount of neurotransmitter moving between brain cells by preventing it from being reabsorbed by the cell that released it. They are very effective in moderate or severe depression in which there are problems with sleeping,

Some side effects of tricyclics

- Blurring of vision
- Constipation
- Difficulty getting an erection and in ejaculation
- Difficulty urinating
- Dry mouth
- Effects on the heart (makes it beat fast or irregularly)
- Fits are rare and occur only in people who are prone to them
- Giddiness on standing
- Sweating
- Tremor of the hands
- Weight gain

appetite, agitation, or retardation. They take up to two weeks to start working.

There are many different tricyclic antidepressants. They all work on depression but have other effects too. Some are sedatives—they calm you down—others are not.

If you are anxious and agitated, your doctor will probably prescribe you a sedative antidepressant whereas if you feel slow and tired all the time, your doctor will probably opt for one that is less sedating. Some people taking sedative tricyclics feel drowsy during the day. This can be reduced by taking the whole day's dose at night rather than three times a day. This may also make you sleep better.

If you drive for a living or use machinery, you should take special care when taking antidepressants. Discuss this with your doctor.

Tricyclics are powerful drugs and like all powerful drugs can have side effects. Not everyone gets side effects but if you do, tell your doctor. They can be reduced by starting the medication at a low level and building up the dose. They can also be reduced by changing the tricyclic that you take.

These antidepressants can interfere with many commonly prescribed medications—even over-the-counter cold and allergy medications—so you should consult your doctor and pharmacist before taking anything else.

An overdose of tricyclics can be fatal. If you or any one you know has taken an overdose, seek medical attention immediately. They will usually be prescribed in small quantities and you should talk to your doctor immediately if you have suicidal or self-harming thoughts.

Tricyclic-like antidepressants

Many drugs act just like tricyclics but do not have the three-ring structure and therefore aren't called tricyclics.

- Ludiomil (maprotiline) has four rings. It should not be taken if you have had epilepsy.

- Desyrel (trazodone) has few side effects, although, in men, it can rarely cause an erection that does not go away which requires urgent medical attention.

- Remeron (mirtazapine) is an effective antidepressant but it can cause blood disorders. Patients should consult their doctor if they have a fever or sore

Some SSRIs

Real (generic) name	Trade (proprietary) name
Fluoxetine	Prozac
Fluvoxamine	Luvox
Paroxetine	Paxil
Sertraline	Zoloft
Citalopram	Celexa
Escitalopram	Lexapro

throat or any sign of infection while taking it. It can also increase the appetite and cause weight gain.

Selective serotonin re-uptake inhibitors (SSRIs)

These work in the same way as tricyclics—they stop neurotransmitters being taken back up into the cell that released them. However, they work on only one type of neurotransmitter—serotonin.

They are effective antidepressants. Although they also have side effects, many people find them more tolerable than the side effects caused by tricyclic antidepressants. As a result, they are very commonly prescribed. They are generally less sedative, may be less

Some side effects of SSRIs

- Diarrhea
- Nausea
- Vomiting
- Headache
- Restlessness
- Anxiety

likely to cause weight gain, and do not affect the heart as much as tricyclics. As with tricyclics, caution is necessary in epilepsy and they can cause stomach problems initially. Diarrhea, nausea, and vomiting can occur as can headache, restlessness, and anxiety. These drugs are generally safer than tricyclics even if an overdose is taken, though this can still cause serious harm. Anyone taking an overdose must seek medical attention immediately

One particular drug—Prozac—has featured extensively in the media. It was the first SSRI to reach the market but it works very much like the others. It has been popularized in some best-selling books and is sometimes characterized as the "happy pill." As a result, many doctors are worried about what they see as the over-prescription of this drug to people with mild depression who may have gotten better with lifestyle changes alone. All SSRIs are as effective as Prozac but should only be prescribed after careful assessment with your doctor.

There has been much concern recently about the potential for these drugs to cause suicidal urges. Suicidal feelings are also a feature of some forms of depression. When starting on these medications, it is important that you monitor yourself for these feelings and report any suicidal thoughts to your doctor immediately

Some Monoamine oxidase inhibitors (MAOIs)

- Nardil (Phenelzine)
- Parnate (Tranylcypromine)

Monoamine oxidase inhibitors (MAOIs)

These were the first antidepressants to be developed. They increase the amount of neurotransmitters in the synapse by stopping them being broken down by a substance called monoamine oxidase. Unfortunately, they also work in the rest of the body where monoamine oxidase has some important functions. One is to break down a chemical called tyramine which is contained in a number of foods. Too much tyramine causes high blood pressure and a violent throbbing headache and can lead to a stroke. As a result, anyone who is taking these drugs must stick to a strict diet low in tyramin and carry a card warning of the condition.

It takes two weeks for the body to make new monoamine oxidase and so it takes two weeks for your body to get back to normal after you have stopped taking monoamine oxidase inhibitors. As a result, you have to stay on the diet for this amount of time; if they have not worked, you may not be able to try another antidepressant drug while still on the diet.

There is a newer type of MAOI called RIMA—reversible inhibitor of monoamine oxidase subtype A. There are two types of monoamine oxidase—type A and type B. As RIMAs inhibit only one type, there is less of a problem with food containing tyramine food, so the diet is less strict. However, people taking them must stick to the diet and could be at the same risk if they eat too many tyramine-rich foods. RIMAs block the action of monoamine oxidase but do not destroy it, so the body does not have to make new monoamine oxidase and the effects are "reversible," wearing off a day after stopping the drug.

MAOIs are generally used if a tricyclic or an SSRI has not worked, but some doctors use them from the start in depression with reverse physical symptoms (for example, where someone eats too much or sleeps more than usual) and they may also be used in people who have a form of depression that does not fit into any of the well-recognized patterns.

Other antidepressants
Serzone (Nefazodone)
This works as an SSRI but has fewer side effects on the stomach. It should not be prescribed to anyone with liver disease. It is better at helping sleep than most SSRIs.

Effexor (Venlafaxine)
This is an antidepressant that works like an SSRI. It sometimes causes an increase in blood pressure, so it should be used with caution in people with high blood pressure. It can cause a skin rash and this should be reported to a doctor immediately because it may indicate a serious allergic reaction. Like many antidepressants, it may affect the performance of skilled tasks, such as driving.

Wellbutrin (buproprion)
This is an effective antidepressant. In high doses, it carries a risk of seizures so it is important not to combine it with other medication without first checking with your doctor. It should not be taken be anyone who has a seizure disorder.

Thyroid Hormones: Cytomel (Liothyronine), Levothroid, Synthroid (Levothyroxine)
Thyroid hormones are used in the treatment of people whose thyroid gland is underactive. They may also be

used in conjunction with other antidepressant treatments for people with depression that is difficult to treat.

Cymbalta (Duloxetine)
This is a new antidepressant that works as an SSRI and is similar to reboxetine in inhibiting the uptake of noradrenaline (norepinephrine). The manufacturers hope that its two-pronged attack on depression will make it more effective.

St. John's wort
Hypericum perforatum (St. John's wort) is a popular herbal remedy for depression, although based on the current evidence it is not generally recommended for more severe depression. Ongoing research is examining the possible role of St. John's wort in the treatment of milder depression. You can buy it without a prescription but it is important to remember that it is quite a powerful herb and can interact with other drugs that you may be taking for depression or physical conditions. Other herbal supplements frequently used that have not been evaluated in large-scale clinical trials are ephedra, ginko biloba, echinacea, and ginseng. Any herbal supplement should only be taken after consultation with your doctor.

Antidepressants and sex
When they are depressed, many people do not feel like having sex. This is part of the depression. However, problems with arousal and ejaculation can also be a side effect of some antidepressant medications. If you are having any such problems you should speak to your doctor. Many people who are depressed suffer in

Stopping antidepressants

Antidepressants should not be stopped without taking professional advice because withdrawal symptoms may occur.

General words of advice

- Do not stop antidepressants suddenly—they should be gradually be tailed off over at least a month; consult your doctor first.

- Some people who have taken antidepressants regularly for weeks and stop suddenly suffer withdrawal symptoms.

- Withdrawal symptoms can be avoided if the dose of antidepressant is gradually reduced over at least four weeks.

Discontinuation symptoms

- Dizziness, electric shock sensations, anxiety and agitation, insomnia, flu-like symptoms, diarrhea, nausea, abdominal pain, tingling of the fingers, mood swings, feeling blue.

Changing antidepressants
This should be done by a doctor. Some antidepressants should not be taken at the same time—they are potentially lethal in combination. You have to let all of one antidepressant leave your system completely before you start another one—this may take between one and five weeks, depending on which antidepressant you are stopping and which you are starting.

silence, but psychiatrists are aware of the side effect and it can be treated.

Mood stabilizers

These drugs are rarely used to treat depression; they are used to prevent it from returning if you are prone to it by keeping your moods stable.

Lithium (Eskalith, Lithobid)

Lithium makes our cells and our moods more stable. People who have bipolar disorder (manic–depressive illness) are less prone to breakdowns if they take lithium. It also prevents depression in people who suffer severe recurrent depression. It can stop relapses altogether or make them shorter and less severe with longer intervals between them.

It has to be taken regularly and has to be at the right level in the blood. Too little does not work and too much causes side effects and can be life-threatening. The amount of lithium that needs to be taken by any individual can be worked out only by blood tests.

Before starting lithium, blood tests will be taken to make sure that your kidneys are working normally and that the chemicals in your blood are correctly balanced. You will be examined and a heart trace will be taken to make sure that your heart is working normally. The action of your thyroid gland will also be tested. If there is evidence of disease of the kidneys or of the heart you may not be able to take lithium.

Once you start lithium, blood tests will be taken at least once a week until the dose settles and then every month for three months. After this, doctors differ: some take blood tests every two months, others less regularly.

Anything that could make you seriously dehydrated, such as going on vacation to a tropical climate, diarrhea, vomiting, or starting a new drug—water tablets, for instance—may alter the amount of lithium that you need to take. A blood test will have to be performed urgently.

If you are to have an operation you should tell the doctor that you are on lithium because it may have to be stopped.

Side effects

Side effects of lithium therapy may include tiredness, more frequent urination, a fine tremor of the hands, a dry mouth, and a metallic taste in the mouth. Many of these disappear with time. These side effects should not be confused with signs that the level in your body is too high. If you have severe shaking of the hands, weakness, diarrhea, vomiting, and confusion, see your doctor or visit the emergency room urgently. You may be suffering from lithium toxicity.

Long-term side effects include weight gain and lithium can also sometimes affect the thyroid gland. As a result of this, some of the blood taken to test the level of lithium will be sent off for thyroid hormone checks a couple of times a year. Low thyroid hormones can be treated by stopping the lithium or by giving thyroid hormone tablets.

Lithium can affect the way that your kidneys function if you have been taking it for a while. It can cause you to urinate frequently and give you a terrible thirst. If this happens, you should see your doctor as you may have to stop taking the medication.

Lithium in pregnancy

Lithium can harm the growing fetus in the early stages of pregnancy so anyone who is on lithium and plans to become pregnant should see their doctor and arrange to stop taking it.

You can start again after three months because the placenta offers some protection to the fetus and the fetus will be less sensitive to it, but this must be done under the supervision of a doctor. The lithium level must be monitored closely because the amount that is needed will change as the pregnancy progresses. More blood tests will be needed than usual.

After birth, the baby is no longer protected by the placenta; lithium gets into the breast milk and can affect the baby, so women on lithium cannot breast-feed.

Carbamazepine (Tegretol)

This is another mood stabilizer. It can be used with lithium or instead of lithium in people who cannot take lithium for one reason or another. Blood tests are performed at least every two weeks for the first two months, and less frequently thereafter. Fever may be an indication of blood problems caused by carbamazepine, so you should consult your doctor if you experience such difficulties.

Sodium valproate (Depakote, Depakene)

This is a drug that is used for epilepsy and has mood-stabilizing functions. In the past, it was used only if neither lithium nor carbamazepine could be given, but now it is the preferred drug of some specialists. Blood tests should be performed regularly.

Other mood stabilizers

Psychiatrists use drugs that are used in brain conditions such as epilepsy, and which have been shown to have a mood-stabilizing action. These drugs are generally used only if more common treatments such as lithium, sodium valproate, and carbamazepine are ineffective.

Other treatments prescribed for depression
Sleeping pills

Problems with sleep are common in depression. They may result from the depression itself, but this is not always the case. Possible other causes for poor sleep, such as a medical problem or perhaps even a tablet prescribed for a medical problem, should be dealt with.

Stress management and other techniques (see page 52) often help sleep. If the sleep problem is the result of the depression, it will improve with antidepressant treatment. If sleeping problems are troublesome, an antidepressant should be chosen that has a sedative action, as well being as an antidepressant.

Sometimes it is not possible to prescribe a sedative antidepressant and, if this is the case, a doctor may prescribe an antidepressant and a sleeping pill. Sleeping pills should be used only for a short time—two weeks at most. Some people find them difficult to stop, become dependent on them, and they may suffer withdrawal symptoms. Even if prescribed for only a short time, they are best used intermittently.

There are many kinds of sleeping pills. Drugs such as Restoril (temazepam) are sometimes prescribed—they are from the same family as Valium (diazepam). There are newer sleeping tablets, such as Ambien (zolpidem) and Sonata (Zoleplen) that work in a similar way to

Valium and also carry a risk of dependence. They should be prescribed for short periods and reviewed regularly by your doctor. Antihistamines such as Benedryl (diphenhydramine) are sometimes used as sleeping aids.

Anti-anxiety pills

Many people with depression also feel anxious. This is a symptom of the depression and, much like sleep, it gets better when the depression gets better.

If anxiety is severe, doctors may prescribe an antianxiety drug with the antidepressant. There are many drugs that are used to treat anxiety, for instance propranolol, Valium (diazepam), Buspar (buspirone), Ativan (lorazepam) and Xanax (alprazolam). However, an antidepressant alone often does the trick as can an antidepressant together with psychological treatments. If an antianxiety drug is to be prescribed in depression, it should be used only in the short term and be carefully monitored by your doctor to avoid the risk of dependence.

For a fuller discussion of anxiety, see the Family Doctor Book *Understanding Anxiety and Panic Attacks*.

Treatment of psychotic depression

People with severe depression may lose touch with reality and develop delusions and hallucinations. In such cases, psychiatrists may prescribe two drugs:

(1) one that has an effect on the depression

(2) one that has an effect on the delusions and hallucinations (an antipsychotic).

Studies have shown that a tricyclic antidepressant and an antipsychotic work better than an antidepressant alone in these cases. Antipsychotic drugs, such as Thorazine (chlorpromazine), Telazine (trifluoperazine) and Haldol (haloperidol), are very powerful and can have a number of severe side effects. Newer antipsychotics, such as Zyprexa (olanzapine), Risperdal (respiridone) and Seroquel (quetiapine) have fewer side effects and are being used by most psychiatrists as the first choice.

Antipsychotic drugs will usually be prescribed only to control the psychotic symptoms and will then be reduced and stopped, leaving the person on the antidepressant alone.

Which antidepressant should I take?

There are many antidepressants on the market. Different doctors often have a preference for one antidepressant based on their own experience. Current research studies show that, in mild to moderate depression, there is little to choose from among the SSRIs, tricyclic, and related antidepressants with regard to their effects on symptoms.

The choice of antidepressant often depends on other things, for instance, whether a particular drug suits you or whether you have had successful treatment or treatment failure before, if a blood relative has had been successfully treated on a particular drug, or if there are problem side effects.

A full discussion with your psychiatrist will help you to make the best choice for your treatment.

Does the drug suit you?

Different antidepressants have different side effects and different people are vulnerable to different side effects.

You will need to inform your doctor of all side effects you experience so that a decision can be made whether to change the drug or not.

Physical problems such as a heart, liver, or kidney condition can influence which antidepressant you can be given. You should remind your doctor of any medical condition that you have, so that you will be offered a proper choice of drug.

The use of antidepressants in pregnant or breast-feeding women requires careful consultation with a psychiatrist to balance the risks and benefits of treatment for the mother and the baby.

Past treatment
If you have had depression before and it has been successfully treated with an antidepressant, it is usually a good idea to try the same one. If it worked before, it will probably work again.

If an antidepressant of one class (for instance, SSRIs) is taken at the correct dose for the correct time and it fails to lift the depression, you might be prescribed a different class of drug (for instance, a tricyclic antidepressant). Changing to another drug from the same class can also sometimes work.

What happens if you have taken two different antidepressants and they have not worked?
Most people get better if they take the first antidepressant that they are given in the right dose for long enough. The remainder usually get better on the second drug that they are given. A minority of people do not get better even after they have been given two

different drugs. If this happens to you, do not despair. There are many alternatives, including:

- using high doses of particular antidepressants
- taking another tablet that boosts the function of the antidepressant that you are taking
- taking a combination of antidepressants.

KEY POINTS

- Antidepressants are an effective treatment
- Antidepressants are not addictive
- Side effects can be lessened by starting with low doses or using newer antidepressants

Physical treatment

Electroconvulsive therapy

Electroconvulsive therapy (ECT) is one of the most controversial of psychiatric treatments. It is also one of the most effective. It works, and works quickly, in the vast majority of people when it is properly prescribed. It has also proven to be safe.

ECT is usually offered to people:

- whose depression has not responded to antidepressants
- who have medical conditions that mean they cannot take antidepressants
- who are so severely depressed that they are endangering their own life (for instance, by not eating or drinking at all).

Some doctors offer it to women with very severe postnatal depression because it starts working straight away and means that they can get back to bonding with their baby.

Some people who have had ECT before and on whom it works well have it as an outpatient but most people stay in hospital as an inpatient.

The idea of convulsive therapy frightens some people. There have been many inaccurate reports that it causes permanent problems in the brain. Although these reports have been disproved, the distrust of ECT remains. ECT has been shown to be a safe and effective treatment. If it did not work and did not work well, it would not be used. Psychiatrists are doctors whose duty is to their patients. Much research has been done into how ECT works but at the time of writing, no one knows how ECT works. Of course, this is the case with many treatments that doctors give for all sorts of illnesses that they do not fully understand.

Studies have shown that ECT does not cause long-term brain problems. Some people have complained of some temporary memory loss, but modifications in the way ECT is given have reduced this. Most people have no memory loss at all and nearly everyone finds that their memory improves as their depression lifts.

ECT cannot solve any underlying problems that caused the depression but it returns the patient to a state in which he or she can start tackling these problems. Like taking drugs for depression, ECT will not guarantee that you will stay well. If you have serious depression you are at risk of a further bout.

What happens in ECT?

An anesthetist gives you a short-acting anesthetic to help you sleep and something to relax you. Oxygen is given by facemask while you are asleep. A small electric current is passed through your brain using electrodes placed on the scalp. The amount of current given is

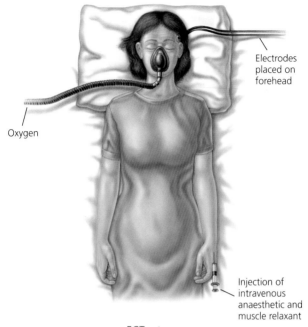

Electrodes placed on forehead

Oxygen

Injection of intravenous anaesthetic and muscle relaxant

ECT set-up.

one-tenth that which is used to start someone's heart if it has stopped. If no anesthetic or muscle relaxant were administered you would have a short fit but because of the anesthetic all that is seen is some twitching of the toes which lasts a few seconds. This is an indication that the brain has a fit but the body does not. You will wake up 10–15 minutes later. Some people complain that their memory is not so good or they feel slightly confused straight after ECT.

ECT starts to work straight away; most people feel significantly better after a couple of weeks. Most people have six to ten treatments over the course of a few weeks (two to three treatments a week).

Getting ECT

Patients and families are often apprehensive about ECT and your psychiatrist will take time to explain the procedure and its effects. Informed consent is needed for ECT just as it is for an operation, and there will be a full discussion with the opportunity to ask questions. You will usually be offered written information and videos that help explain the process so that you can study them at your own pace. If you do not consent, ECT will not usually be administered. It is very rare for ECT to be given against the patient's will and then only in cases where treatment is urgent, for example if the patient is not eating or drinking, and with the consent of family or a legally appointed guardian. The treating psychiatrist will be familiar with the local, state, and federal laws governing ECT.

Transcranial magnetic stimulation

Repetitive transcranial magnetic stimulation is a new technique that some believe could be useful in the treatment of depression. A very strong, pulsed magnetic field is produced from a hand-held baton that is held against the head. Initial studies have shown that it is safe and useful. However, more studies are needed before it can be recommended.

KEY POINTS

- ECT is given only to people who desperately need it

- It is a safe treatment for depression

- ECT does not lead to brain damage

What happens when you visit your doctor?

If you think that you are suffering from depression, your primary care physician may be the first person whom you should consult. Most managed care insurers require you to see your primary care physician before you can be referred to a psychiatrist. He or she will be able to offer experienced help:

- Your primary care physician will discuss your problems and make sure that they are not the result of a physical illness.

- Your primary care physician will make an initial assessment of the severity of your depression.

- If you have mild depression, you may not be prescribed medication. You may be given advice and/or offered psychotherapy or counseling, and your primary care physician will see you again to make sure there is an improvement.

- If you have moderate depression, your primary care physician may offer to start you on an antidepressant medication before recommending psychiatry, although it is more likely he or she will want you to see the psychiatrist first. He or she may also refer you for psychotherapy or counseling.

- If you don't want to take antidepressants you should still keep your appointment with the psychiatrist as he or she will be able to discuss the alternatives, risks, and benefits with you and monitor your progress. You should also carefully consider your psychiatrist's advice if he or she thinks that you need medication. Talk it over with your family and friends. If necessary, you could ask for a second opinion from another psychiatrist.

- If you have severe depression, your primary care physician will refer you for an urgent appointment with a psychiatrist. This will depend on your symptoms. If you have symptoms such as suicidal thoughts he or she will send you to the emergency room for immediate evaluation.

- If you are prescribed medication, your psychiatrist will want to see you a week or two after starting the antidepressants. This is to make sure that you do not have side effects and can take the tablets.

- If you cannot tolerate the drugs they can be changed—so tell your doctor if you have problems.

- Medication works gradually; sleep and tiredness may improve first—depressed mood often takes longer.

- You will see your psychiatrist regularly to get more medication and to make sure that things are going well. If you are receiving psychotherapy from a therapist other than your psychiatrist, he or she will usually ask for your written permission to talk with your therapist so that they can both monitor your progress.

- After about six weeks, most people feel much better. All your symptoms may not have gone, but you will be well on the road to recovery. You should continue to improve over the next few weeks.

- Even though you feel much better, you should continue to take your medication for another six months or so. Your psychiatrist will monitor you to decide the safest time to stop the medication. After this you will come off them slowly, not all at once.

- If you have not improved, your psychiatrist may increase the dose and may want to see you more frequently.

- If you have not improved even though you have been taking the medication as prescribed, your psychiatrist will be able to suggest alternative medications or treatment strategies such as dosage adjustments. Sometimes a different medication is all that is needed. Sometimes a different class of medication is needed. Very rarely, combinations of medications may be used. Your psychiatrist may also consider sending you to a specialist psychopharmo-cologist (a psychiatrist who specializes in the use of medication) for a second opinion

- If your situation worsens your psychiatrist may suggest you go into hospital for further assessment.

- If nothing else works and you are very depressed you may be offered ECT.

- If you are severely depressed from the outset—deluded, suicidal, or not eating and drinking—your psychiatrist will arrange hospitalization so that treatment can be started in a safe environment.

Staying well

Once you have recovered from an episode of depression the challenge is keeping well.

Those who have had one bout of depression are at higher risk of having another bout than those who have never suffered from depression.

There are, however, many ways of decreasing the chance of another bout:

- Gradually try to increase the activities that you enjoy
- Take regular exercise—it helps your mood
- Avoid alcohol and illegal/leisure drugs, both of which can make you feel depressed once the initial effects wear off
- If you feel isolated but do not want to feel a burden to your friends, join a self-help group to talk through your problems and feelings
- Use the relaxation techniques in this book whenever you feel stressed (see page 54)
- If you have been in therapy, try to make sure that you use the problem-solving and communication skills you were taught
- Two to four top-up sessions of brief psychotherapies, such as cognitive–behavioral therapy, over a 12-month period may decrease the chance of relapse
- Take the medication that you are prescribed for as long as is recommended without missing any
- If you have had one bout of depression you may be recommended medication for six months to a year; if you have had more than one bout of depression you may be advised to stay on medication for at least two years
- If you have recurrent episodes of depression, your doctor may recommend you start taking a drug called lithium, that has been proved to reduce the number of episodes of depression that people get
- If you decide you want to stop or reduce the dose of your medicine, do this only after discussing it with your doctor

Women and depression

Depression and gender

Women are twice as likely as men to be diagnosed with depression. There are a number of possible reasons for this:

- It may just be a reflection of the fact that women are more likely to admit to their feelings than men.

- It may be that male doctors see women as being prone to depression and so diagnose it more often.

- It may just be a reflection of the fact that women go to the doctor more often than men, so doctors have more chance of diagnosing depression.

All of these are important factors but there are also physical differences between men and women that seem to make women more prone to depression. The most important of these is the levels of the sex hormones estrogen and progesterone. Women have a higher level of these hormones and the levels change during the menstrual cycle, throughout pregnancy and childbirth, and at the menopause. Oral contraceptive containing sex hormones can be a cause of depression.

Menstrual cycle

Levels of progesterone and estrogen vary through the menstrual cycle. Progesterone is produced on average for only 10 days before menstruation and then its level drops. It has been implicated as a cause of premenstrual syndrome or PMS that usually begins a few days before the start of menstruation and usually ends shortly after the onset of menstruation—some symptoms of PMS stop as soon as the period begins.

Not all women have the same combination of PMS symptoms, but tender breasts, feelings of distension and abdominal discomfort, together with irritability, anxiety and depression, are particularly common. It is important to distinguish premenstrual syndrome from premenstrual worsening of a depression.

Although many treatments have been used for PMS, including hormone therapy and water-reduction tablets (diuretics), they often do not work very well. Physical exercise and psychotherapy (especially cognitive behavioral therapy) have been shown to be helpful in some cases. Support, sympathy, and understanding will also help in most cases. Antidepressant treatment is given only to people with severe symptoms.

Depression and motherhood

The levels of estrogen and progesterone are very high in pregnancy and drop dramatically after the baby is born; this sudden change can sometimes trigger depression. About half of women experience the maternity or baby blues, 15 percent get mild to moderate postnatal depression and one in 500 experiences severe postnatal depression.

Maternity blues
Half of new mothers suffer from "maternity blues" in the week after the birth. It's usually around about the third day after the birth that a new mother may start to feel irritable and weepy. Usually she will be back to her old self again by the end of the first week and all she needs in the meantime is support, love, and understanding.

Mild and moderate postnatal depression
Long-term depression is common after childbirth. It often goes unnoticed as it is put down to the new

mother adjusting to her responsibilities or being kept awake at night by the baby. The severest types of depression occur soon after the birth of the baby but the least severe and most common start between two weeks and a year later. Sometimes they may start around the time when the support and attention of friends and family start to wane. The symptoms may be less specific than in other types of depression. Often the woman is very anxious, especially about whether her baby is well and feeding properly, and she may seem to be full of guilt and self-criticism as well as constantly tired and irritable.

Postnatal depression cannot be explained simply by hormone changes. For one thing, the major changes in hormone levels often occur long before the depression begins. They may make a woman prone to depression but social factors are important too.

In general, women are at increased risk of postnatal depression after a particularly difficult pregnancy or birth, when the reality of motherhood or the change in role fall below expectations and/or when having a new baby brings relationship difficulties to the fore.

Treatment is usually needed for postnatal depression. A recent study showed that both antidepressant drugs and cognitive–behavioral therapy (see page 66) are effective. Most antidepressants can be taken while breast-feeding.

When a woman is being treated for postnatal depression, it usually helps if her partner can become involved and understand the problem. In some cases, fathers may be in need of support too; there is a high risk of depression in new fathers who have depressed partners. Treatment makes a big difference to recovery rate. Women who are treated for postnatal depression

The risk factors for postnatal depression

Certain factors increase the likelihood of the new mother suffering from postnatal depression. The more risk factors a woman has, the greater her chance of depression.

Before the baby is born
- Fertility problems
- Past psychiatric illness
- Psychiatric illness in the family
- Single parent
- Serious financial problems
- Having a child when very young (under 16 years)
- Having a child when over 35 years of age
- Uncertainty whether you want the baby
- Worries about the baby's health
- Mild-to-moderate anxiety during the last three months of pregnancy
- A difficult labor

After the baby is born
- Pre-term birth (delivery before week 37)
- Physical illness
- Social isolation
- Lack of support from your partner
- Returning to work at a lower level of seniority

are likely to recover completely, whereas those who don't have a 50:50 chance of feeling better by the child's first birthday.

Severe postnatal depression

A more unusual type of postnatal depression affects a minority of women who become severely depressed in the first four weeks after the baby is born. It is more likely:

- after the first pregnancy
- in those who have had a psychiatric illness before
- in those who have psychiatric illness in the family.

It is thought that hormonal change may act as a trigger for depression in those who are prone to it.

In severe depression, a woman loses touch with reality and she may have delusions and hallucinations. This is considered a psychiatric emergency and typically requires hospital treatment as there is a real risk to the mother and her baby in this situation. The ideal place is a hospital mother-and-baby unit, where she can be with her baby and have help from the staff to care for him or her.

Treatment is usually with antidepressants and she may also have other types of medication to deal with hallucinations and delusions. The mother may be recommended to stop breast-feeding because of possible effects of medication in breast milk on the baby. The doctors will be able to discuss the risk/benefit balance of a particular medication in detail. A mother who is being treated with lithium (see page 83) will be recommended to stop breast-feeding as babies are very sensitive to its effects.

Some doctors offer electroconvulsive therapy (ECT) for severe depression after childbirth when medications fail or it is imperative to get a rapid result. It works quickly and enables the new mother to continue bonding with her child. The vast majority of women are treated with medication.

If you have had postnatal depression you are likely to make a good recovery but you will be at risk of developing it after any future pregnancies. You should tell your doctor or obstetrician that you have had postnatal depression before you have your next baby so that you can be monitored and receive early and prompt treatment if you need it.

The menopause

Although women are more likely to seek help for depression around their middle years, there is no reliable evidence that depression is actually more common at the time of the menopause.

There are, of course, a number of other changes that happen in many women's lives in middle age which may be playing a role in triggering depression. For example, children leave home, the relationship with their partner may change, and their own parents may become ill.

It is possible that hormone changes during this time also affect a woman's vulnerability to depression. Hormone replacement therapy (HRT) is relatively often prescribed to treat menopausal symptoms and some women say that they also feel less depressed while taking it. Women who have a depressive illness and happen to be around the time of the menopause can also be treated with antidepressants if appropriate, just like anyone else with a similar condition.

Hysterectomy and sterilization

Research from some years ago claimed that women were more likely to become depressed after either being sterilized or having a hysterectomy, but recent research has cast doubt on this. The ovaries produce a number of hormones whose functions are unclear and some doctors have suggested that, in some women, their removal will cause depression. Other doctors say that hysterectomy triggers depression only in a woman who is already predisposed to psychiatric illness, while some experts point out that there are some women who actually recover from psychiatric symptoms after a hysterectomy.

The same applies to sterilization operations. In other words, it may only be those women who were at risk of depression anyway who will become clinically depressed after being sterilized.

Women at home

Women may have a higher rate of depression because of their social situation rather than due to their hormones. Some women become isolated because they are alone at home during the day. One study of women at home found that the most likely people to be depressed were young mothers with three or more children under the age of ten, with an unsupportive partner, no one else to confide in, poorly housed, and having no employment outside the home.

KEY POINTS

- There are many reasons why women are diagnosed with depression more often than men

- Changes in estrogen and progesterone may trigger depression

- Depression after childbirth is often missed but can be treated effectively

Depression in young people

Symptoms of depression in young people
There are many similarities between depression in children and depression in adults but there are also important differences.

Many of the symptoms of depression are the same in young people as they are in adults. As with adults, there is a change in mood that persists over time. There are physical symptoms such as poor sleep or too much sleep and low energy levels, and there are psychological symptoms such as poor concentration, and a negative view of the world and their place in it.

However, many young people will deny feeling sad even though their behavior has changed, and they have become grumpy or irritable. There is no consistent way in which depression in children shows itself. Some young people come to the attention of the family physician or pediatrician because they complain of headaches, stomach pains, or bone pain but no cause can be found. Others present for the first time with self-harm, disinterest in general appearance, withdrawal, and loss of interest, but in others a change in behavior such as a decline in schoolwork or increased argumentativeness is the first sign.

Symptoms of depression vary according to age. Children are more likely to complain of physical problems such as headaches and abdominal pains and tend not to look depressed. Adolescents are more likely to complain of feeling blue and to have a higher rate of suicidal thoughts.

Moody or depressed?

Surveys have shown that many young people have some depressive symptoms but they are not serious enough to be considered an illness or need treatment.

Trying to disentangle depression from normal mood problems in teenagers can be difficult. One indication is that depressed teenagers often no longer derive pleasure from life and have poor self-esteem. They may have little to say when asked about their good points, they think that they are no good and that the situation in which they find themselves is their fault, but they do not have the ability to change things. When this is coupled with the adult symptoms of depression, such as poor concentration, loss of confidence and, in severe cases, delusions and suicidal thoughts, the diagnosis is not too difficult. In this situation you should contact your doctor immediately.

Depressive illness is diagnosed when the symptoms lead to significant personal suffering and social impairment.

It often takes time to make the diagnosis. As with adults, many young people are not forthcoming when seeing a doctor or therapist. As with adults, depression can also be considered as mild, moderate, or severe, depending on the number and intensity of symptoms that are present.

One rule of thumb is that depression needs treating only if it stops someone from doing what they want or changes their ability to do things, for instance, if it interferes with their schoolwork. In any case, you should talk to your primary care physician or pediatrician in the first instance if you have concerns and they will help you find a psychiatrist.

Risk factors and figures

Depression is less common in young people than it is in adults. Each year approximately one percent of pre-pubertal children and three percent of post-pubertal adolescents suffer from depression.

Some of the underlying causes of depression in children are similar to the causes for depression in adult life, for instance genes, personality, or family environment. Others, such as bullying, being placed in foster care, personality, social development in adolescence, changes in hormones, and brain development, are specific to young people.

More than 95 percent of major depressive episodes in young people arise in children and young people with long-standing difficulties, such as family or marital disharmony, divorce and separation, domestic violence, physical and sexual abuse, school difficulties, and exam failure.

A very small number of depressive episodes in children and young people will arise in the absence of prior difficulties, and result from an acute life event such as a mugging.

Depression is triggered by an event that has a high negative impact, for instance parental separation or getting into relationship difficulties with a close friend.

Social stress seems to be an important underlying factor because the rates of depression are higher in families with social problems such as poverty.

Depression in children and young people can often occur in conjunction with other mental health problems such as abuse of drugs or alcohol or hyperactivity.

Treatment of depression in childhood

Many young people who are depressed do not get treatment. This is because they are reluctant to seek help as a result of the stigma of mental health problems, but they also do not get help because depression is missed by parents, health professionals, and teachers. Depression may be missed in three-quarters of young people who suffer from it.

Treatment strategies should be aimed at the whole child. Many young people with depression suffer from

Some high-risk groups for childhood depression

- Those who refuse to go to school
- Abused children
- Young people who have experienced a significant traumatic event
- Young people who repeatedly harm themselves
- Young people in chronic family disputes
- Young people with persistent drug and alcohol problems.

other mental health problems and there are often social and family issues, so everything has to be dealt with. Attention should be paid to the possible need for treatment of the parents' own psychiatric problems, such as depression.

A treatment program should aim to:

- cure the depression
- improve other mental health problems
- improve social and emotional development and school performance
- decrease family distress
- reduce the risk of relapse.

Treatment for depression in the young can involve many different people who should all be aware of the young person's needs and the treatment plan. These may include the primary care physician, pediatrician, teachers, school nurses, clinical child psychologist, social workers, educational psychologists, child and adolescent psychiatrists, child and adolescent psychotherapists, counselors, and family therapists. More severe depression may also require the services of a child and adolescent psychiatry day unit or highly specialized outpatient teams and inpatient units.

Most young people with depression are treated in the outpatient setting. Only a few are ever hospitalized in a specialist inpatient unit.

Mild depression

Most pediatricians and family doctors will refer young people with depression to a child and adolescent psychiatrist for an initial assessment. A psychiatrist will give the patient the opportunity to be seen alone as well as with a parent. If the depression is diagnosed as being mild depression the sort of treatment that might be offered would include:

(1) individual supportive psychotherapy

(2) group cognitive–behavioral therapy

(3) guided self-help (see box below).

Antidepressant medication is not generally used for the initial treatment of children and young people with mild depression.

Moderate-to-severe depression

If an assessment reveals complicating factors, for instance significant risks such as suicidal thoughts, mental health problems such as substance misuse or mental health problems in other family members, the psychiatrist will consider whether inpatient treatment is necessary and will also recommend a higher level of

Guided self-help for mild depression

Guided self-help should include:

- Books and educational leaflets about depression
- Advice on the benefits of regular exercise and a supervised exercise program (three sessions a week lasting 45 minutes through 1 hour for up to three months)
- Advice on achieving good quality sleep and anxiety management
- Advice on nutrition and the benefits of a balanced diet

treatment such as a specific psychotherapy, for example individual cognitive–behavioral therapy, interpersonal therapy or family therapy. Additional therapy on a one-to-one basis for the young person or parents may be considered.

Given the complex and serious nature of depression, a number of professionals may be involved, each trying to improve a specific aspect of the problem. For instance, in addition to a psychiatrist, educational psychologists may be helping with school, family therapists with family difficulties, and social workers with financial, housing, or legal problems.

Medication

If psychological therapies are not effective, doctors may consider adding medication to the treatment. Antidepressant medication should be offered only in combination with psychological therapies. If psychological therapies are refused antidepressants can be prescribed alone but there needs to be close monitoring—preferably weekly for at least the first four weeks. This is because side effects need to be assessed and because in some young people there is concern that antidepressants make them feel more suicidal.

In those aged over 12 there is some evidence that one drug—Prozac (fluoxetine), an SSRI (selective serotonin release inhibitor)—is effective. In the five-through 11-year-old age group the evidence that any drug is effective is sparse. For this reason, the use of antidepressant medication in the treatment of children is controversial although many doctors feel that the benefits are sufficient to outweigh the risks when the child is severely depressed. This is a decision that needs

Antidepressant treatment in children

- Antidepressants should be offered only in combination with psychological therapy
- Antidepressants should be prescribed in low doses
- Antidepressants may be given if psychological therapies are refused but there should be close monitoring of mood and side effects
- Antidepressants should be prescribed only after assessment and diagnosis by a child and adolescent psychiatrist
- Antidepressants should only be prescribed only after a full discussion with the child and adolescent psychiatrist and a decision that, in the individual child, the benefits outweigh risks
- All antidepressants must be monitored for side effects and for the possible development of suicidal thoughts
- Antidepressants should be continued for approximately six months after symptoms have disappeared, depending on the individual situation
- Medication should be stopped slowly over a 6- to 12-week period
- St. John's wort can interact with antidepressants and if a young person is taking them they should be advised to stop.

to be made on an individual basis after an informed discussion with your psychiatrist.

Admission to hospital
Admission to hospital must be considered if the child/young person is at high risk of suicide, serious self-harm and self-neglect, the required intensity of treatment (or supervision) is not available in the community, or intensive assessment is needed.

Once depression has resolved
A young person who has suffered from depression is at increased risk of another bout. As a result, a psychiatrist will usually keep an eye on the person for at least a year after the depression has resolved. In addition, a psychiatrist will be able to respond quickly them if symptoms return.

What is the outlook?
Depression in children is a serious illness. While many recover in time without treatment, treatment can decrease the duration and severity of the illness.

The most serious complication of depression is suicide—three percent of depressed children kill themselves within the next ten years; other problems are poor school performance and difficulties in personality development. One in three young people with depression experiences a recurrence within five years and many develop episodes into adult life. Prompt recognition of the problem is essential to access adequate health care.

KEY POINTS

■ Many of the symptoms of depression are the same in young people as they are in adults

■ Depression in young people is often triggered by an event that has a high negative impact—for example, parental separation

■ Treatment for depression in young people can involve multiple professional from different backgrounds

■ Antidepressant medications are not be used for the initial treatment of young people with mild depression

Grief and bereavement

The link between bereavement and depression

There is a complex link between bereavement and depression. Bereavement can trigger a depressive illness, though it usually does not. However, a recently bereaved person can experience many symptoms that are similar to depression. In one study, about 30 percent of recently bereaved widows over the age of 62 were found to meet the criteria for depressive illness.

In bereavement, suicidal thoughts, mental and physical slowness, and worry about past actions are much less likely to occur. If you suffer from these you may be depressed, rather than just grieving, and treatment may be needed. If you have thoughts of self-harm or completely stop eating you should see a doctor urgently.

Normal grief

Grief is a normal experience; it is painful but does not need medical treatment. There are three stages.

1. Numbness
This lasts from a few hours to one week. You may feel emotionally numb and feel as if the person hasn't died or that you can't accept the reality of their death.

2. Mourning
From one week to six months (easier after about three months). You may feel sad, depressed, have little appetite, find yourself crying a lot, or be agitated, anxious, and have little concentration. Some people feel guilty. They feel that they had not done enough for the deceased. Others blame professionals, friends, and family. You may find that you have physical symptoms, such as pains, during this phase.

Most people have the feeling at some time during this stage that the deceased is present in some way and one in ten report either seeing, hearing, or smelling the dead person when they are not there. Many of the experiences mimic depression but they are normal—you are not depressed or going mad.

3. Acceptance
Six months onward, the symptoms subside. You start to accept the death and try to get back to normal. This takes a variable amount of time.

Coping with grief
Grief is natural and so are your feelings. Grief is a process that has to be worked through. If it is not, then feelings could fester and they could catch up on you in later life, turning into depression. Grief should not be bottled up and needs to be let out.

Even if you seem to be having a severe reaction to the death at first, you are likely to come through the process with just the support of your friends and family or a counselor.

It is usually best to turn to your family and friends initially. They will all need to grieve themselves and the help and support they offer you will help them to come to terms with what has happened. You are not a burden, it is a two-way thing. They need you as well.

Counselors can offer support in grief and can help people work through the process in a controlled way. They are particularly useful if you find that you are not passing through the stages of grief or you are having a particularly difficult time. Bereavement counselors aim

Causes of intense grief

Although the death of a loved one is always hard to bear, certain situations make the grief even more intense:

- If the death is sudden or unexpected
- If the death results in blame for the survivor
- When a parent's child dies
- When a young child's parent dies
- When an adult was dependent on the person who died
- When the survivor has difficulties expressing his or her feelings
- When the survivor is currently still adapting to a previous loss
- When the survivor is socially isolated
- When the survivor has dependent children

to help you acknowledge the death by helping you talk about the circumstances surrounding it; they encourage the emotional expression of the pain of grief; they try to identify coping strategies and people who might offer support; they help the process of building a new life and help you let go of the dead person. You can contact such counselors through your primary care physician, local psychiatric service, or call the psychiatric hotline, listed under "Useful information," page 136.

Supporting someone who is grieving

Giving space for a grieving person to talk about their feelings is all important. Most people think that they need to say how wonderful the deceased was but that is often not the support that someone needs:

- They need space to talk about how they feel.
- They need to be allowed to say;
  - how bad they feel.
  - how distressed they are.
  - how they might feel guilty.
  - how they feel angry that they have been left behind.
  - how they said something bad before the person died.
  - how the death brings their own mortality closer.

All these thoughts and feelings are normal and need expression.

Medication

Medication can be counterproductive early on in the grieving process. Though drugs may make you feel better they may interfere with the process of grieving and prolong it. It is painful to work through the feelings of loss but it is the only way to get back to normal.

If you really cannot sleep at all for the first few days your doctor may prescribe tranquilizers. This will only be for a few days to help you sleep and then they will be stopped. In extreme circumstances these may be useful for a few critical days but should not be used long term. Though they may help you to feel better they will not help you work through your grief and you will have to do this when you stop taking the tablets. It is only if grief turns into depression that drug treatment has any place long term.

Self-help
A number of self-help organizations can offer advice and support. For a listing of some of them see "Useful information" on page 133. These are national organizations, who will advise you of your local or state organizations, or you can look these up in the phone book or on the internet.

Abnormal grief
Not everybody passes through the stages of grief smoothly. Some people find that they do not pass through the normal stages and suffer persistent problems. Others find it difficult to grieve and do not acknowledge the death at all. Some people find that they are consumed with intense anger or feelings of betrayal that last for months. If grief is intense and unbearable it needs to be treated. Contact your primary care physician or a counselor.

KEY POINTS

- Grief is a normal reaction

- Medication is not usually needed and may be counterproductive

- Self-help organizations provide excellent bereavement counseling

Helping friends and family

The value of talking and listening

If you are able to recognize when someone is depressed and offer support, your help will be priceless. You may not think that you have done very much but you will have helped someone in need and may even have helped prevent a suicide.

Many people who are depressed find it difficult to take up offers of help so don't be put off. Try to be patient and tell them that you are ready to talk when they want to.

When you talk, be sympathetic, be supportive, and try to convince them to see their primary care physician or a psychiatrist. There is no point telling a person who is depressed to snap out of it or to pull themselves together. Nobody likes being depressed and they would snap out of it if they could.

Talking allows people to work through their problems, but listening is not easy. It can be uncomfortable, especially when someone you know is distressed and they are saying things that are either not true or so painful that you do not know how to cope with the emotions that they produce in you. Do not take on too much.

Try not to give quick ungrounded reassurance or quick advice and don't think that you have to say something because you feel uncomfortable. Do not jump in and interrupt—give them time and space to say what they feel. Accept that they feel the way they do and see the world the way that they do. If you think that they are wrong, explain why you think so and give them proof, but do not get into an argument. You will be doing a good job if you listen, acknowledge how the person feels, be sympathetic, and hold back on giving too much advice.

Remember, you can assure them that medical treatment is effective and that they will get better.

Once you have talked things through, try to keep in touch, be accessible, and offer practical help and support until they are better. Helping people to get help by offering to accompany them to a doctor's appointment can be useful but be careful not to take over. Many people with depression feel ineffective and taking over their decisions may make them feel worse.

Preventing suicide

Suicide is a leading cause of death in the United States accounting for more than 30,000 deaths each year. Most people suffering from depression get better. The box on page 131 lists groups of people who are at high risk but it should be borne in mind that anyone who is seriously depressed may be thinking about suicide and you should be vigilant.

Attempts at suicide are not just a way of getting attention and they should always be taken seriously. Of course, there are people who try to harm themselves as a cry for help—but if that cry goes unheard, goes wrong, or is in the context of a depression, then it could herald suicide.

Knowing about depression, ensuring that someone who is depressed gets treatment, and keeping in touch are important.

Supporting someone who is suicidal without professional help is very difficult. If you are at all worried you should try to convince the sufferer to see someone as soon as possible. They can go to their primary care physician, the hospital emergency room, or see a local psychiatrist. Your local psychiatric department may have an emergency clinic that you can just walk into.

Helping a friend who is suicidal

If you suspect that a person is suicidal, talk with them and let them speak about their feelings. Ask them if they have ever thought that it was not worth going on with life. Some may say "yes" and that they have thought of taking their own life; others may say that they have not thought of it but they have gone to bed at night hoping that they would not wake up. Both groups of people are potential suicide risks. Of course some people intent on suicide will deny that they have thought of it; you may have to make a judgment as to whether they are telling the truth. Many people find speaking about their suicidal impulses is a tremendous release and it may actually make them less likely to go through with it.

Tell them they need to see someone urgently and that help is available. They will probably agree that they should see someone, but if they do not and you really think that they are a danger to themselves, you should act in their interests. The quickest way to get help is to call the emergency services. You can contact the local psychiatric department and see if there is a walk-in clinic. You can take them to an emergency room.

If you can get their agreement to remove Tylenol and any antidepressant or non-essential drugs from their medicine cabinet, this would be a good move.

If you are worried that your friend is in imminent danger do not leave him or her while you are getting in contact with helping agencies if at all possible.

It is always best to discuss what you are doing with the sufferer. You may also want to contact their family.

If you feel suicidal—seek help. Speak to someone urgently.

Factors that increase suicide risk

The likelihood of a person committing suicide is increased if any of the following conditions or categories applies:

- Severe depression
- Serious physical illness accompanying depression
- Person has spoken about suicide
- Past suicide attempt
- Suicide in the family
- Continuing severe life stresses such as divorce or bereavement
- People who are lonely and socially isolated
- Men, who are more likely to succeed in their suicide attempt
- Unemployed individuals
- People taking illicit drugs
- Those with alcohol problems

KEY POINTS

■ Listening may be the most important thing that you can do for family and friends who are depressed

■ Anyone who thinks about suicide should contact their family doctor, psychiatrist, emergency room at the local hospital, or the psychiatric hotline, and get help

■ Depression can be treated—you will feel better

Useful information

Where can I learn more?

We have included the following organizations because, on preliminary investigation, they may be of use to the reader. However, we do not have first-hand experience of each organization and so cannot guarantee the organization's integrity. The reader must therefore exercise his or her own discretion and judgment when making further inquiries.

Resources specific to depression

Hotline Numbers

National Suicide Prevention Lifeline (800) 273-TALK

National Drug and Alcohol Treatment Hotline (800) 662-HELP

National Domestic Violence Hotline (800) 799–7233 or (800) 787-3224

National Child Abuse Hotline (800) 4-A-CHILD

National Youth Crisis Hotline (800) HIT-HOME

National Runaway Switchboard (800) 621–4000

Panic Disorder Information Line (800) 64-PANIC

Project Inform HIV/AIDS treatment Hotline (800) 822–7422

American Psychiatric Association
1000 Wilson Blvd
Suite 1825
Arlington VA 22209
(703) 907–7300
www.healthyminds.org

Depression and Bipolar Support Alliance (DBSA)
730 N. Franklin Street
Suite 501
Chicago IL 60610–7224
(800) 826-3632
www.dbsalliance.org

National Alliance for the Mentally Ill (NAMI)
Colonial Place Three
2107 Wilson Blvd
Suite 300
Arlington VA 22201–3042
(703) 524–7600
Information Helpline: (800) 950-NAMI (6264)
www.nami.org

National Mental Health Association (NMHA)
201 N. Beauregard Street
12th Floor
Alexandria VA 22311
(800) 969-NMHA (6642)
www.nmha.org

General information resources
Freedom From Smoking® Online
www.ffsonline.org

American Lung Association's free online smoking cessation program.

Healthfinder®
www.healthfinder.gov

A consumer health information website sponsored by the United States government. A resource for finding government and non profit health information on the internet.

National Health Information Center (NHIC)
P O Box 1133
Washington, DC 20013
U.S.A.
Tel: (800) 336–4797
www.health.gov/NHIC

NHIC, part of the Department of Health and Human Services, helps people locate information on health issues through referral to organizations that can best answer their questions.

U.S. Department of Health and Human Services
200 Independence Avenue, S.W.
Washington, D.C. 20201
Tel: (202) 619–0257
Helpline: (877) 696–6775
www.hhs.gov

Government agency giving information and advice on sickness and disability benefits for people with disabilities and their caregivers.

Further reading

Depression: The way out of your prison, by Dorothy Rowe, Routledge, 2003.

Breaking the Bonds: Understanding Depression, Finding Freedom, by Dorothy Rowe. HarperCollins, 1996.

Malignant Sadness: The Anatomy of Depression, by Lewis Wolpert. Faber & Faber, 2001.

The internet as a source of further information

After reading this book, you may feel that you would like further information on the subject. The internet is, of course, an excellent place to look and many websites contain useful information about medical conditions, related charities, and support groups.

It should always be remembered, however, that the internet is unregulated and anyone is free to set up a website and add information to it. Many websites offer impartial advice and information that has been compiled and checked by qualified medical professionals. Some, on the other hand, are run by commercial organizations with the purpose of promoting their own products. Others still are run by pressure groups, some of which will provide carefully assessed and accurate information whereas others may be suggesting medications or treatments that are not supported by the medical and scientific community.

Unless you know the address of the website you want to visit—for example, www.webmd.com—you may find the following guidelines useful when searching the internet for information.

Search engines and other searchable sites
Google (www.google.com) is the most popular search engine used in the United States, followed by Yahoo! (www.yahoo.com) and MSN (www.msncom). Also popular are the search engines provided by Internet Service Providers such as AOL (www.aol.com).

In addition to the search engines that index the whole of the web, there are also medical sites with search facilities, which act almost like mini-search engines, covering only medical topics or even a particular area of medicine. Again, it is wise to look at who is responsible for compiling the information offered to ensure that it is impartial and medically accurate.

Search phrases
Be specific when entering a search phrase. Searching for information on "cancer" will return results for many different types of cancer as well as on cancer in general. You may even find sites offering astrological information! More useful results will be returned by using search phrases such as "lung cancer" and "treatments for lung cancer." Both Google and Yahoo offer an advanced search option that includes the ability to search for the exact phrase; enclosing the search phrase in quotes, that is, "treatments for lung cancer," will have the same effect. Limiting a search to an exact phrase reduces the number of results returned but it is best to refine a search to an exact match only if you are not getting useful results with a normal search.

Always remember the internet is international and unregulated. It holds a wealth of valuable information but individual sites may be biased, out-of-date, or just plain wrong. Family Doctor Publications accepts no responsibility for the content of links published in this series.

Index

Your pages

We have included the following pages because they may help you manage your illness or condition and its treatment.

Before an appointment with a health professional, it can be useful to write down a short list of questions of things that you do not understand, so that you can make sure that you do not forget anything.

Some of the sections may not be relevant to your circumstances.

Health-care contact details

Name:

Practitioner type:

Place of work:

Tel:

Name:

Practitioner type:

Place of work:

Tel:

Name:

Practitioner type:

Place of work:

Tel:

Name:

Practitioner type:

Place of work:

Tel:

Significant past health events – illnesses/operations/investigations/treatments

Event	Month	Year	Age (at time)

Appointments for health care

Name:

Place:

Date:

Time:

Tel:

Name:

Place:

Date:

Time:

Tel:

Name:

Place:

Date:

Time:

Tel:

Name:

Place:

Date:

Time:

Tel:

Appointments for health care

Name:

Place:

Date:

Time:

Tel:

Name:

Place:

Date:

Time:

Tel:

Name:

Place:

Date:

Time:

Tel:

Name:

Place:

Date:

Time:

Tel:

Current medication(s) prescribed by your doctor

Medicine name:

Purpose:

Frequency & dose:

Start date:

End date:

Medicine name:

Purpose:

Frequency & dose:

Start date:

End date:

Medicine name:

Purpose:

Frequency & dose:

Start date:

End date:

Medicine name:

Purpose:

Frequency & dose:

Start date:

End date:

Other medicines/supplements you are taking, not prescribed by your doctor

Medicine/treatment:

Purpose:

Frequency & dose:

Start date:

End date:

Medicine/treatment:

Purpose:

Frequency & dose:

Start date:

End date:

Medicine/treatment:

Purpose:

Frequency & dose:

Start date:

End date:

Medicine/treatment:

Purpose:

Frequency & dose:

Start date:

End date:

Questions to ask at appointments
(Note: do bear in mind that doctors work under great time pressure, so long lists may not be helpful for either of you)

Questions to ask at appointments
(Note: do bear in mind that doctors work under great time
pressure, so long lists may not be helpful for either of you)

Notes

Notes

Notes

Notes

Notes

Notes

Notes

Notes

Notes

Notes

Notes

Notes

Notes

Notes

Notes